# Restoring America's Health

## *Simple Steps to a Plant-Based Lifestyle*

### By: Chef Nancy A. Stein

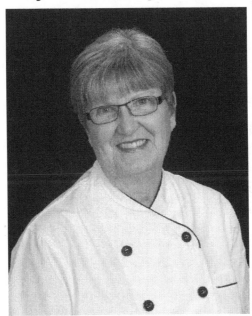

*Cover Photograph, Courtesy of Plant Based Road Trip*
http://plantbasedroadtrip.com

*Cover Design inspired by Daniel R. Peek*
http://daniel.peekent.com

# *Dedication*

This book is dedicated to beloved family members who have passed away from our number one killers in America today: Heart Disease, Type 2 Diabetes, and Cancer; and to our 7 grandchildren who I hope to inspire healthy lifestyle choices, so as not to experience these dreadful complications with preventive health care that starts with good food choices. I love you, and to my husband Skip, the love of my life who inspires and encourages me daily to believe in myself and not be afraid of life's challenges, I love you.

## In Memory

Father Homer (Heart Disease)
Mother Hazel (Bladder Cancer)
Sister Barbara (Arteriosclerosis)
Sister Mary (Heart Disease/Lung Cancer)
Father-in-law Henry (Prostate Cancer)
Brother-in-law Don (Diabetes)
Brother-in-law Bob (Pancreatic Cancer)
Mother-in-law Bernice (Arteriosclerosis)

### *YOU ARE LOVED AND MISSED*

# Medical Disclaimer

This book is not intended to diagnose, treat, cure, or prevent any disease. The information and opinions contained in this manual do not replace or substitute for the advice of a practicing medical doctor. Please consult your physician before beginning any new diet, supplement regimen, or exercise program. The author disclaims any and all responsibility for the information in this book in regard to current health conditions such as heart disease, allergies, diabetes, cancer and auto immune diseases. Again, please check with your doctor before embarking on any new diet. The author shall not be responsible for any loss or damage suffered by you, the reader, or anyone else in connection with this book or the information contained in it. Please do not discontinue taking any prescribed medications without the consent of your doctor.

The information presented in this book is founded on the author's opinion and belief and is based on experiential evidence from the author's life.

# Table of Contents

# Restoring America's Health

# Restoring America's Health

## Background & Introduction

In 2016 the oldest Baby Boomers began turning 70 years of age, myself and my husband included. We don't actually feel different at age 70, but aging has made us contemplate just how short life is, as we see so many of our family members and friends passing away from dreadful diseases that seem to be expected as we age: cancer, heart disease, diabetes and more. Research has shown that these diseases are not age-related but created by *poor lifestyle choices*. These illnesses used to be called "senior diseases"; they were expected to happen, but now are striking every age, as our Standard American Diet high in fat, sugar, and sodium are now contributing to sickness, disease, and ill health in all Americans. Research today confirms that consuming a diet high in animal-based foods and processed foods vs. plant foods is detrimental to our health and causing us to be sick.

This book is a guide to help you understand that our day to day choices in life can either help us maintain healthy living as we age, or can develop into life-shortening illnesses and disabilities. It is a guide to inspire everyone to consider their present lifestyle and help you enact healthy changes into your life. You will find the recipes provided at the end of this book easy to prepare and will enable you to jumpstart your personal goals to become healthier and happier in life by eating whole foods, exercising, and reducing daily stress.

## Welcoming Change into Our Lives

Implementing a lifestyle change isn't easy, but can be achieved by taking simple steps, such as eating healthfully, hydrating, moderate exercise, and finding time alone with ourselves. How often do you step outside and breathe deeply, while sensing all the beauty that surrounds us and is completely free for the taking?

**No Cellphones, No Computers, No Worries about our pending "To-Do Lists".**

Simple changes like this can begin a new stage in our lives providing overall health and wellness, inner growth, peace, and renewal. A simple step like solitude, time alone with ourselves helps us to reduce stress in our lives. It can awaken our senses that perhaps have been dormant for years and held us back from achieving a heathier you. It may be just finding time in our day or maybe just *fear*, but either way, both lack of time and fear can prevent us from attaining healthy goals.

Achieving change, whether positive or negative, allows us to continually re-evaluate our lives and see things from a different perspective. We have the option to fix what is ineffective and not working, but we must first accept, recognize, and be open to change in order for the fix to benefit and improve our lives. Not all changes are equal some may bring happiness and others sadness. Change makes us strong in who we are as a person and allows us to deal with all situations in life.

If we stay stuck in our routine lives, we become stagnate, predictable, and uninteresting. Today we live in a fast-paced modern-day world. Life in general becomes so robotic it has a tendency to become comfortable as is for most Americans. Lifestyle changes can be a challenge; however, it can be an opportunity and exciting journey for everyone to experience if you want to live a life free of the things that hold us back, make us ill, and prevent our lives from moving forward. There will always be bumps along the way, such as sudden change, which can happen at any point in our lives as it did for me and my husband's lives.

## Our Story

Our story begins in 1995; it was a difficult year in my life. My mother was ill with bladder cancer and the prognosis didn't look good. I was juggling work and being a caregiver for my mother and never realized stress was building up inside me and would soon become my worst enemy for my own health. I started to get severe pain in my right hip and it became more and more pronounced. It was becoming difficult to sleep at night and walk the next day. I thought to myself that it was nothing and that I had probably just pulled a muscle. Each day the pain began to migrate further until it encompassed my entire body. Too painful to sleep, sit, or stand too long, inflammation was everywhere in my body and that made every movement and every touch unbearable.

I began to visit numerous doctors and went through several procedures to rule out MS, Lyme's disease, rheumatoid arthritis, and lupus. Still, the doctors had no answers for me. Their best prescription was prednisone medications for pain and muscle relaxers to sleep at night. Nothing seemed to work and symptoms only got worse and even more debilitating.

The prescription medications caused weight gain, which in turn, aggravated my symptoms even more. Four years of testing and medications went by, when finally, fibromyalgia entered the picture. It was unknown and undiagnosed back then, and blood tests could not identify this illness. Doctors tested painful trigger points on your body; if you had all 18 you were diagnosed with fibromyalgia. So finally, I was getting some answers and I felt relieved, but treatments didn't work and my pain progressed along with sleepless nights attributed to a lack of REM sleep, another common side effect of fibromyalgia. This lack of sleeping soundly created a feeling of brain fog throughout my day along with other challenges that continued to happen, such as chronic fatigue syndrome and Epstein Barr virus, each taking their toll on my health.

I was exhausted and went to work in severe pain and came home to severe pain 24 hours a day. I finally succumbed to the illness and realized I would have to live this way the rest of my life, as doctors basically said there was no cure as they continued to treat my never-ending list of symptoms with prescription drugs. It was difficult being around family and friends, as I knew they were thinking and often saying I was a hypochondriac. They could see I looked great on the outside, but found it difficult to understand my chronic fatigue and the pain I was experiencing on the inside. This only brought more stress and affected my ability to perform everyday activities as though nothing was wrong.

Back then I didn't have the internet to conduct research. I had to find out answers from the few books on the market that talked about fibromyalgia. I soon realized stress, sleep, and diet were the #1 factors.

In 1999 the illness took yet another toll on me. I had an anxiety attack at work (another common side effect of fibromyalgia) and I decided to take early retirement from a position I loved working, knowing that this would be the best thing for my health and sanity. I still continued under my doctor's care and included chiropractic treatments, but again, nothing really changed. I was at a dead end for answers and suffered from 1995 until 2010.

2010 brought about another stressful twist and turn in my life. My husband came home from the doctor's office and was diagnosed with aggressive prostate cancer. I was devastated over the news and unclear where to turn or what to do, (all I could think about was that his father had recently passed away from the same dreadful cancer and how quickly chemotherapy took his life).

My husband's prognosis for living was 3 years, maybe 5 with conventional treatment, a combination of surgery, radiation, and chemotherapy; very bleak to say the least. Our lives were turned upside down. The doctors wanted him to make his decision on treatments that day, but fortunately my husband decided to go home and digest all that was being recommended.

We began to research all the available information online. We discovered that our bodies have the miraculous power to heal, if given the proper nutrition. Thinking about that cut or bad burn that healed quickly, we learned that our own natural immune system was the key to healing. We knew we had to take steps to get his immune system working at peak level. This is when our lifestyle change began.

Knowledge is everything and it's available to us in several ways: in books, on TV, and on our computers. You can research just about any topic online and find an answer: however, look closely as to where the information and research is coming from. We found several research articles on prostate cancer and found a common thread from articles written by T. Colin Campbell who wrote *The China Study*, Dr. Neal Barnard from the Physicians Committee for Responsible Medicine, and Dr. Michael Greger, M.D. who scours the world's nutritional research papers for the latest up to date information on all medical issues. We watched a TV program called *The Incurables*, where people who were diagnosed with stage 4 cancers were sent home to die but instead made a lifestyle change and cured themselves. We asked ourselves, how can this be? Why haven't we heard this from our doctors? We became so intrigued and wanted to learn more. Our research found the common thread was simply **lifestyle change. Diet and nutrition** became the answer.

The common thread was food—whole food. We had to begin eliminating bad food choices that included highly processed foods and foods that were genetically modified along with foods that were high in saturated fat and cholesterol, hydrogenated oils, high fructose corn syrup, soda and just plain junk foods. We needed to be on a **whole foods plant-based diet.**

No meat, fish, dairy, eggs, or derivatives found in highly processed foods. Our own research taught us that animal protein was linked to cancer and plant proteins healed. We decided at that moment diet change was needed and that it was a lot cheaper and less painful than surgery, chemo, and radiation with **NO** debilitating side effects.

Overnight we changed our diets. We gave away (with guilt) all our processed foods, meat, fish, and any products that contained dairy or eggs to remove any temptations. I bought a vegan cookbook to learn how to cook a plant-based diet and our journey began. It was a huge step for us and a surprise to our family. They were a little distraught with our decision to believe that food would be the prescription to make us healthy again. We believed so confidently in our research that we wanted to take this challenge to see what would happen.

I admit to being scared that my husband might die; but this acted as a strong incentive to begin a lifestyle change. We did have some challenges getting used to this new way of life. After all, we, too, were brought up eating these very foods that were high in saturated fat and cholesterol and realized that our previous lifestyle had contributed to all our current health issues!

We began our journey with about a three-month body cleanse: juicing greens and vegetables to help rid our bodies of food-borne and daily environmental toxins while at the same time learning to prepare our meals with whole grains, beans, vegetables, and greens. We soon realized how delicious our food began to taste. In thirty days, we began seeing results in weight loss, which continued over the course of 6 months I had lost 85 lbs. and my husband lost 50 lbs. My husband's total cholesterol was 148 and although not perfect yet, my cholesterol came down from 243 to 170 and my LDL went from 195 down to 119. Our blood sugar was normal, no more acid reflux (I had taken over the counter medications daily), and our energy levels spiked. Most doctors can tell you there are no medications that can perform this well in 30 days. My husband's PSA went down, not up, and my fibromyalgia was disappearing. I couldn't stop thinking why anyone wouldn't want to embrace this great feeling of wellness and even consider returning to our Standard American Diet high in fat, cholesterol, sugar, and salt. I guess that's why many refer to our Standard American Diet as the "SAD" diet.

Unfortunately, there is no magic pill for health and wellness. The perfect prescription is consuming whole foods, not artificial foods. Whole foods provide our bodies with all the nutrients they require for optimal performance. Only a whole food plant-based diet can provide this and dramatically improve our immune system to fight off disease and not promote disease.

Eight years have passed and we still have more energy than we know what to do with. We are 70 and don't take any medications. My husband's health is amazing (he still gets his yearly checkup at the doctors as do I). And remember how I couldn't walk, stand or sit too long? Well, we have since begun hiking and have been traveling around the USA, seeing all that we can see and enjoying new adventures.

Life is about choices we make for ourselves. We all make mistakes in life, but we can correct our mistakes and move forward with better decisions. The word cancer is just that, a word and yet a blessing, as it gave us a big wake-up call. We would probably be dead by now had we both continued on the devastating path eating whatever we desired, not exercising, and not taking responsibility for our own health and wellness. We became empowered when we invited **change** into our lives. We changed our lifestyle and fully embraced a whole new world of living instead of dying.

## Paying it Forward

I re-entered school in 2012 and earned my Certificate in Plant-Based Nutrition from the T. Colin Campbell Foundation through e/Cornell University, mainly to learn more and more about the benefits of a plant-based diet. It was, and continues to be, my sincere desire to pay it forward and encourage others to experience the benefits a whole food plant-based diet can provide; not only for themselves, but for their entire family's health and wellness.

Preventive care is key and unfortunately most people live their lives treating their symptoms, but not the cause of their ill health and never get well. Preventive care and a proper nutritional approach can do just that: prevent us from getting ill in the first place. Unfortunately, people today are so used to waking up with a headache, sinus infection, and overwhelming fatigue that it makes it difficult to just get through their day. As a nation, we have forgotten what it's like to really feel well. We hear over and over again from people who say they are just tired of being sick all the time.

I have been teaching how to begin a whole foods plant-based diet and cooking classes for eight years now. My students are from all walks of life, different ages, and include both healthy men and women, and those challenged with newly diagnosed health issues, heart disease, diabetes and even cancer. Achieving the benefits of a healthy lifestyle only works if you are open to change and want to live a lifestyle with optimal health and wellness for yourself and that of your family. It's by no means a diet where today we eat healthy and tomorrow we eat whatever we want. It's taking charge of our health on a daily basis for the rest of our lives.

Teaching about a plant-based lifestyle has opened our eyes to not only understanding how to eat a healthy diet, but also realizing, from talking to others, what makes changing one's lifestyle so difficult. Let's face it, most of us have been eating whatever we want without having to think about health consequences. TV advertisements and misleading information provided by magazines and the internet, tell us one day something is good for us and the next day it isn't. All of this misinformation and struggling to stay healthy has only made people yo-yo diet, spending large amounts of money on this pill or supplement that promises quick results in weight loss and good health, but only gives you a temporary fix, not long-term health benefits.

It's amazing that today you can even buy supplements that are extracts from whole fruits and vegetables. Supplements in pill extracts will never compare to the nutrients in the actual whole fruit or vegetable and they are by far more expensive than buying whole foods.

I have heard every excuse as to why someone can't or won't change their lifestyle. Many blame their spouse or children as not wanting to follow a healthy diet. Others say they just can't live without their steak and would rather die. Some are just, well, tired juggling job and family that they find cooking just too demanding. It's often much easier to eat out or pop a meal in the microwave. Many say it's in our family genes: my mother, my father, my sister or brother had it, so I am bound to have it as well. Then you hear it's too expensive to buy beans, vegetables, and fruit; yet we find a way to buy a new smart phone or latest gadget or fashion. It really does come down to choices in life. Some will be good choices and others well, not so good, and sadly for some it may be too late.

You have to think "change" for yourself first. An addiction of any kind is hard to break and you may be surprised to hear that food is addictive for many people. Processed foods and fast food create a "pleasure trap" for us, as these foods are high in fat, cholesterol, sugar, and salt and are meant to be addictive and keep us coming back for more and more. The "Big Food Giants" know this and want us coming back to buy their products, not caring whether it makes us sick or not. It's hard to break this cycle of unhealthy foods and you will find you won't change everyone's mind in your family at first to make the same healthy decisions as you want to make, but when they see positive results that you are having with a healthy lifestyle they will become more aware and more apt to want the same change in their lives.

I have met so many wonderful people teaching plant-based nutrition who inspire me every day. Their fight, their courage, their spiritual, emotional, physical, and mental outlook prove that you can either take a back seat to life's challenges or be in the front seat taking charge of your own health and wellness and living life to its fullest. It's a fact we are all going to die, but we are talking about *quality of life* until the end. Life doesn't have to end being immobile or hooked up to machines that keep us alive for a few more days or months.

I realize not everyone is going to read this information and change their diet overnight, but I hope it will at least bring *health awareness* to you. When you pick up that candy bar or soda drink you might question whether this

19

food is doing something good for your body and if not, replace it with food that is alive and wholesome.

Research on the benefits of eating a plant-based diet has already been done for you by leading doctors and scientists and they have produced not only books on health and wellness, but inspiring health documentaries available on Netflix (also available to purchase on DVD), such as, *Forks Over Knives* and *A Delicate Balance, Eating You alive* and *What the Health*. These documentaries have provided health awareness and changed people's lifestyles dramatically.

This book is about **our** choices and may not be for everyone, and that is fine, but I hope for many that you at least try making small changes in your diet which are better than no changes at all. The more you consume whole foods rather than highly processed foods and foods that are high in saturated fat and cholesterol (like meat, fish, dairy, and eggs) the more you will find renewed health and wellness. I hope with the help of this book I can offer encouraging hope to others who maybe suffering from heart disease, type 2 diabetes, cancer, or other autoimmune diseases and see for yourself if a whole foods plant-based diet doesn't offer you renewed energy, hope, and wellness.

A quote from Charlotte Gerson from the Gerson Institute (GersonInstitute.com): *"You can't keep one disease and heal two others - when the body heals it heals everything."*

Following a plant-based lifestyle includes several other alternative and holistic aspects that keep our bodies in balance spiritually, mentally, emotionally, and physically. Consuming healthy foods, hydrating our bodies properly, and engaging in moderate exercise should be a daily practice. Holistic approaches such as meditation, aromatherapy, yoga, tai chi, are activities that bring harmony and balance to our bodies and support the elimination of daily environmental and food-borne toxins we are exposed to on a daily basis. There are several alternative and holistic approaches to heal many of our common day-to-day ailments that you may want to try. Chiropractic care, massage therapy, application and use of essential oils and acupuncture are among the many alternative and less invasive treatments available today to fight illness and disease. Research has shown them to be highly effective in healing our bodies and moving us forward to health and wellness. Everyone has the potential to live long, healthy, and happy lives. We can avoid many of the side effects from invasive treatments and pharmaceutical drugs by practicing preventive care and not waiting until illness and disease strike first.

It doesn't matter if your choice of treatment is alternative or conventional medicine. What does matter first and foremost is our diet: the number 1 treatment option which may make all other treatment decisions perform even better.

Research is so important and your doctors seldom have the time to do this or are not capable to answer your questions about nutrition. Most doctors have had no more than a few hours of education, if that, on nutrition and most eat the same unhealthy Standard American Diet as other Americans. It is up to each and every one of us to find our own answers that may provide us better options in our own health care. Whether one chooses conventional treatments, alternative treatments, or a combination of both, you are taking charge of the decision-making in your own life and not relying on others to do this for you.

Our story is just one of many. Our journey just one of many and our life's challenges just one of many. For some, reading our story may find hope. For others, this may revive a special memory of a family member or friend who faced similar challenges in life, but unfortunately, never heard of the power of a plant-based diet as medicine.

Remember you can choose to live a healthy lifestyle or remain captive of the food manufacturers, pharmaceuticals, dairy and meat industries. Even negativity from family and friends can make transitioning to a healthier lifestyle difficult. I ask you today to take this challenge to embrace CHANGE for yourself first. In doing so, you will be a better person, a happier person, and a healthier person, which will then resonate with all your family and friends.

Remember it's not important if others follow you and you may find you even lose friends, but realize you will also gain new friends who are like-minded in health and wellness and will support your goals. It's your body, your health, and time for *you!* You can make a difference one step at a time. Do not fear change; embrace change and others will want to follow!

# Wishing You and Your Family Health and Wellness

Chef Nancy

# Health Check

## Check with Your Doctor

It is highly recommended anyone changing their diet to first and foremost have a complete physical checkup with their doctor and notify their doctor of their planned dietary change. To stay on top of your health, consider a physical checkup once a year. It is surprising how many people have no idea where their health stands. Do not stop taking any medications your doctors have prescribed. You need to work with your doctor as a whole foods plant-based diet is a powerful diet. Committing to a whole foods plant-based lifestyle could affect the dosage needed for any condition and as time progresses, you may no longer need some (the same level or any) of the medications currently being taken. Understanding these steps will make your transition to eating a whole foods plant-based diet safer and more successful.

It's important to know and understand the following:

- Your Total Blood Cholesterol
- Cholesterol Ratios
- Vitamin D3 Level
- B-12 Level
- Blood Sugar Count
- Thyroid
- Blood Pressure
- Kidney Function
- Liver Function
- Stress Test
- Women: Breast Mammogram
- Men: PSA (Prostate test)

Additional testing you may want your doctor to perform:

- **Abdominal Ultrasound Test**: This test is a simple ultrasound that can check for a number of conditions. It may be used to screen for an abdominal aortic aneurysm which is a weakened, bulging spot in your abdominal aorta. This artery runs through the middle of your abdomen and supplies blood to the lower half of your body. It is recommended for men age 65-75 and who are current or former smokers. According to the Mayo Clinic if you have never smoked this test is not a requirement unless your doctor suspects an aneurysm could be present.

- **C-Reactive Protein (CPR) Test**: Checks inflammation in the arteries and one's risk for heart disease. C-reactive protein (CRP) is a substance produced by the liver in response to inflammation. Other names for CRP are high-sensitivity C-reactive protein (hs-CRP) and ultra-sensitive C-reactive protein (us-CRP). A high level of CRP in the blood is a marker of any condition that causes inflammation, from an upper respiratory infection to cancer. High CRP levels can indicate that there is inflammation in the arteries of the heart, which can mean a higher risk for heart attack.

- **IGF1:** Insulin-like growth factor (IGF-1) is a natural human growth hormone instrumental in normal growth during childhood, but its presence in adulthood could promote abnormal growth—the proliferation, spread (metastasis), and invasion of cancer.

## Supplements

Many people tend to follow mainstream practices that you need to take supplements daily for optimal health without changing our diets or exercising. When you change to a whole foods plant-based diet many of these supplements can be eliminated as you are now getting these nutrients where they should come from, and that is whole foods rather than from pills.

- **B-12 Supplement**: Vitamin B-12 is a water-soluble vitamin necessary for the maintenance of a healthy nervous system and for the metabolic utilization of fats and proteins. Vitamin B-12 is also essential for the synthesis of DNA during cell division and therefore is especially important for rapidly multiplying cells, such as blood cells.

  A whole foods plant-based lifestyle includes a diet that is powerful and it will provide our bodies with all the necessary nutrients, such as fiber, vitamins, minerals, amino acids, antioxidants and protein, for our bodies to operate at peak level.
  B-12 concerns many people on a strict vegan diet. You will find B-12 in foods such as fortified products, especially in cereals, nutritional yeast and several non-dairy milk options now on the market. If you are concerned about getting enough B-12 in your diet, one of the best options for adequate B-12 is to supplement with a sub-lingual B-12 supplement found at most health food markets, drug stores, and online suppliers. If you prefer a pill, try a Methyl B-12 (as Methylcobalamin) lozenge.

- **Vitamin D3** is often overlooked, but is so important in preventing disease. How do you get Vitamin D3? The best option is being in the sun just 15 minutes a day. You can easily get enough vitamin D3 during your 30-minute walk each day when the sun is not at its hottest. I live in sunny Florida where the sun is abundant year-round, but for those who live in northern and eastern states where sun is not always available, especially during winter months, it is wise to supplement with vitamin D3 during this time until sunny weather returns.

- **Iodine** is often overlooked. I mention this since many on a whole foods plant-based diet may use sea salt which is iodine-free. The good news is you can buy sea salt now with iodine in it, but if you can't find it where you live you can always take an iodine supplement made from sea kelp and is also available in a shaker to sprinkle on your salads or other dishes for added safety. If you are salt-free, then adding a shake of kelp to your salad could be a benefit.

- **Multivitamin:** A high quality multivitamin can be a safety net for any vitamin or mineral deficiency that you may be missing or believe you are missing. It is an inexpensive insurance policy.

## Hydration

Many people today are suffering from dehydration without really noticing it until they actually become thirsty. Signs of dehydration are:

- Increased thirst
- Dry mouth
- Light-headedness
- Fatigue
- Impaired mental focus
- Low urine output
- Inability to produce tears
- Sunken eyes
- Dry skin

The obvious solution to dehydration is to make sure the drink of your day is WATER in place of soda pop, energy drinks (filled with sugar), or other processed bottled liquids. Many physicians recommend a minimum of eight (8) ten-ounce glasses of clean water daily.

## Your Body's PH

Our bodies have numerous mechanisms in place to maintain a pH of about 7.4, or slightly alkaline as opposed to acidic (below 7.0) The closer you are to this ideal mark, the better you feel and the easier it becomes to maintain long-term health. Health issues arise when our pH level becomes acidic or below a pH of 7.0. When your body begins to shift to an acidic environment, this leads to inflammation which affects your whole body. Staying in an acidic environment long-term may contribute to type 2 diabetes, heart disease, or even cancer. Our bodies prefer to be more alkaline and less acidic. Improving your pH level will help in preventing illness and infections which seem to thrive in an acidic environment. Eating a whole foods plant-based diet protects us from being too acidic and maintains a healthy pH level that improves our overall health.

It is easy to test your own pH level with pH strips you can purchase online or from many health-food stores. Test yourself to see if your diet is promoting an acidic or alkaline environment. Consuming animal protein appears to create an acidic environment whereas plant protein creates an alkaline environment.

# What Does Plant-Based Mean?

A plant-based diet is a Vegan diet. No meat, fish, dairy, or eggs. It sounds overwhelming, but trust me, as you continue, you will see how easy it can be to transition away from an unhealthy diet to a powerful, delicious, and healthy diet.

There are lots of myths and misunderstandings of the word "vegan" today and why one may choose to consume a vegan diet. Many are concerned with cruelty to animals and others are concerned for our environment, as raising animals for food requires massive amounts of land, energy, and water. Others are concerned (and rightfully so) in regard to food-borne illnesses from consuming animal-based foods that can threaten our lives daily and cause many to be hospitalized and for some even death.

A whole foods plant-based diet has been shown to be the healthiest way to eat. Not only is it low in saturated fat and zero cholesterol, laboratory research around the world has shown that high amounts of animal protein in our diets may be detrimental to our health causing more heart disease, type 2 diabetes, cancer, kidney disease and more. A plant-based diet is high in fiber and it provides nutrients and antioxidants our bodies need. As plant-based vegans we follow a whole food plant-based diet. We eliminate all meat, fish, dairy, and eggs, as well as most processed foods while striving to keep all cooking oils to a minimum. We now consume whole grains, vegetables, greens, beans and legumes (and other plant proteins like tofu, tempeh and seitan), fruit, nuts, and seeds.

## Cleaning Out Our Pantry/Refrigerator/Freezer

The first step we need to do when changing to a plant-based diet is to remove unhealthy temptations we have lingering on our pantry shelves and in our refrigerator and freezer. Not everyone in your family is going to agree with this lifestyle change immediately; it's important to accommodate everyone's needs to keep the peace in your home. It may be necessary to have a shelf designated with your healthy foods separate from other family members' items making it easier for you to move forward with your goals to be healthy.

A whole food plant-based diet is geared around foods that include beans, whole grains, vegetables, greens, fruit, nuts, and seeds and replacing our meat with tofu, tempeh and seitan. There are also many vegan transitional meat analogues found in most grocery stores today. These meat analogues may provide a bridge to help you transition from an animal based diet to a plant-based diet more easily.

Here is a list of food items you want to **avoid** stocking in your pantry, refrigerator, and freezer that contain unhealthy ingredients. Start by placing all the items from your pantry on a table and consider removing items that have the following ingredients:

- *Enriched* white breads
- *Enriched* bagels (look for whole grain and dairy free)
- *Enriched* English muffins (look for whole grain and dairy free)
- *Enriched* hamburger and hot dog buns (look for whole grain and dairy-free)
- Hydrogenated oils and high fructose corn syrup
- Check ingredient labels when buying frozen pancakes, waffles, and tortillas. Look for 100 % whole grain (organic is possible) with no dairy, eggs, hydrogenated oils, or high fructose corn syrup on the ingredient label.
- White rice
- Food additives and preservatives such as

BHA/BHT, artificial colorings, MSG, nitrates, and artificial flavorings.
- Hidden dairy and animal ingredients such as beef broth, chicken broth, whey, dry milk, egg wash.
- Foods high in saturated fats and trans fat
- Foods high in sodium
- Soda pop of any kind. Choose a healthier beverage such as water or tea. Remember, juices are loaded with sugar and many may contain no real fruit at all.
- Freezer foods to eliminate: All meat and fish
- Refrigerated foods: All dairy (milk, cheese, and butter) and other refrigerated items that contain these ingredients. Remove all eggs.

## GMOs- Genetically Modified Foods

You have all heard the term GMO, which stands for *Genetically Modified Organism*, but what exactly does this mean? The big industry name in GMO is Monsanto. They are considered the mother of agricultural biotechnology. The company produces biotechnology, genomics, and herbicides for corn, cotton, soy, oil seeds, and many other vegetable crops. They produce genetically altered seeds which are then being sprayed with potent chemicals like glyphosate in Roundup, (derived from Agent Orange), and others.

Genetically modified foods are found in most processed foods (unless labeled non-GMO), and on some fresh vegetables and fruit. GMO foods have been shown to cause adverse health effects in many people. A warlike debate has been going on for years asking our government to provide consumer labeling whether a product is GMO or non-GMO and the demand from consumers to label products is there, but in many cases government has done its best to ignore or take their time concerning this issue. Times are changing slowly as more and more products are showing non-GMO labels. It would be better to avoid foods that do not have the non-GMO verification label on them. Buying organic or from our local farmer's market will assure us a healthier life.

## Understanding Food Labels and Labeling

Our pantries should now be cleared from highly processed foods and our refrigerators cleared of dairy and eggs and our freezer free of all meats and fish. This is a step in the right direction. Now you need to focus on reading labels and restocking foods with plant-based ingredients. When shopping, if it comes in a box or bag, look for the non-GMO label. Next, look at the ingredient list. If the list is so long, which many are, and you cannot pronounce most of the ingredients, place it back on the shelf.

Processed foods found on the shelves in your local market contain ingredients such as soy oil, corn oil, and cottonseed oil. If there is no non-GMO verification label on the product, it is possible the product is more than likely to contain those nasty GMOs sprayed with Roundup/Glyphosate. Other ingredients have hidden animal protein in them under tricky names such as "natural flavoring", or may have chicken or beef broth, and don't forget dairy and eggs. For instance, you might see the word "whey" which is dairy, or "egg wash", which of course means eggs are in this product. You can visit "Go Dairy Free" online for a complete list of hidden dairy found in many products and look for the letter "V" or the word "vegan" on products, which assures you this product does not contain animal byproducts.

Minimally processed foods may be bought for flavoring plant-based recipes such as artichoke hearts, roasted red peppers, capers, pickles, olives, canned organic tomatoes (diced, stewed, crushed, whole, paste). The ingredient label should be easy to read with words you can pronounce. For example, a jar of roasted red peppers should state ingredients as roasted red peppers and sea salt. Once you get used to reading ingredient labels you will soon realize, on your own, which labels are considered healthy and what is not.

Make time for your grocery shopping. Avoiding and processed foods you once bought like snacks, cookies, candy, and pastries, can be overwhelming at first and may take you a little longer to shop. It takes practice. If you hurry your shopping or shop when hungry you will tend to fall into the manufacturers' hands and purchase items that are not healthy but *convenient.* It is better to avoid the center aisles where manufacturers play a huge part promoting unhealthy food choices and buyer beware as your local grocery store plays a big role as well when stocking their aisles. Healthy foods tend to be placed high on the shelves and unhealthy foods eye level. Many stores are stocking healthy options alongside unhealthy options making it harder for consumers to identify healthier choices.

## Trans Fat

Trans fat is used in products to enhance and extend shelf life of products. It is found in many processed foods under names such as margarine or partially hydrogenated vegetable oils. Trans fat increases our bad LDL cholesterol and decreases our HDL good cholesterol levels and placing us at a greater risk for heart disease.

## Food Additives

Let's look at food additives. Food manufacturers add many of these food additives to enhance the flavor of their products and to prolong shelf life. Understand and be cautious of additives that may cause addiction to a food and possible adverse health issues.

## Artificial Sweeteners

Aspartame (more commonly known as NutraSweet and Equal) and Sucralose (known as the brand Splenda) are considered by many to be neurotoxins and are carcinogens. These sweeteners should be avoided.

## High Fructose Corn Syrup

High fructose corn syrup has become one of the most problematic foods causing obesity in the United States and promotes type 2 diabetes.

## Monosodium Glutamate (MSG)

MSG is an amino acid used by food manufacturers and restaurants as a flavor enhancer and is an excitotoxin. Regular consumption of MSG may cause severe adverse side effects in many people.

## Common Food Dyes & Colorings

Did you know that food coloring is found in foods such as fruit juices, soda, and salad dressings? Food colorings have been banned in many countries but are still used widely in America. Food colorings have been linked to childhood behavioral problems. Studies have linked food dyes and colorings to cancer. You need to watch out for these food colorings listed on the ingredient labels before buying.

- Blue #1 and Blue #2
- Red dye #3 and Red #40 and E124
- Yellow #6 and Yellow Tartrazine (E102)

## Preservatives

### Sodium Sulfite
Sodium Sulfite is a preservative most commonly

found in wine and dried fruits and other processed foods. Many people suffer from sensitivities when consuming sulfites. It can worsen asthma in some and headaches and rashes in others.

### Sodium Nitrates/Sodium Nitrite

Sodium nitrates are found in foods like bacon, processed lunch meat, hot dogs and corned beef. It is a carcinogen and should be avoided at all cost. You can find many vegan options at your grocery store to replace these foods with plant-based options that include bacon, lunch meat, and hot dogs that are very tasty and avoid these carcinogens.

### BHA and BHT (E320)

Butylated Hydroxyanisole (BHA) and Butylated Hydroxytoluene (BHT) are preservatives used in cereals, chewing gum, potato chips, and in vegetable oils. These preservatives keep foods from changing colors, changing flavors, and provide longer shelf life. These preservatives have the potential to promote cancer.

### Sulfur Dioxide (E220)

Sulfur additives are toxic and are now prohibited by the FDA for their use on raw fruit and vegetables. Read ingredient labels on beer, soft drinks, dried fruit, juices, cordials, wine, vinegar, and potato products.

### Potassium Bromate

Potassium Bromate is an additive used to increase the volume in some white flour, bread, and rolls. This additive is known to cause cancer in humans. Avoid this ingredient.

# How to Read Nutrition Labels

By now you may be feeling a bit overwhelmed, however, my point in all of this information is to bring knowledge to you regarding food you are consuming daily without actually inspecting the ingredient label. This awareness will help you begin to take charge of your health and avoid many illnesses and diseases that are preventable just by reading what manufactures are adding to their products and choosing not to buy a product that is promoting adverse health issues.

## Serving Size and Nutrients

The size and serving on the food package influences the number of calories. One should pay special attention to how many servings there are in the food package to become aware of how many servings you are consuming of a particular product.

- Calories provide a measurement of how much energy you may be getting in a serving from this product. Too many Americans consume more calories than recommended.
- Reduce eating too much fat such as saturated fat, trans fat, cholesterol, and sodium that may increase your risk of certain chronic diseases such as heart disease, cancers, and high blood pressure.
- Check fiber content, as most Americans do not get enough fiber in their diets. Check for 3g or more of fiber on a package serving. Check vitamin content in the product you are buying. Does it have Vitamin A, C, calcium, and iron? Keep sugars low.

This labeling must appear on all packaged or processed food. The Percent Daily Value (%DV) on the Nutrition Facts label is a guide to the nutrients in one serving of food and are based on a 2,000-calorie diet, however, the remaining information only appears if the label is long enough. Each nutrient listed is a DV or %DV providing dietary advice or a goal. Following these guidelines will enable you to know that they are within public health experts recommended upper or lower limits for the nutrients listed, based on a 2,000-calorie diet.

## Nutritional Information

Switching from an animal-based diet to a plant-based diet such as whole grains, beans and legumes, vegetables, fruits, and leafy greens, eliminates our intake of excess fat, cholesterol, sodium, and sugar while providing our bodies with the necessary nutrients to keep us healthy and well. Everyone new to this type of eating may be asking how we get our protein, calcium and healthy fats into our diet. Let's take a look...

### Protein

Protein can be found in whole grains, beans, lentils, tofu, and tempeh. Seitan is another option. Seitan is a meat alternative that can either be homemade or purchased at your supermarket and is offered by companies like Gardein, Tofurky, Lightlife, Field Roast, and Beyond Meat, who offer meatless analogues that resemble chicken, beef, turkey, fish, and pork entrees. We refer to these as "transitional foods". These food products help us transition from an animal-based diet to a plant-based diet. As you become more experienced with plant based cooking you will find many recipes online and in cookbooks that offer great recipes for creating your own meatless analogs as well. Protein is also found in nuts (almonds and walnuts) and seeds and may surprise you that vegetables such as broccoli, spinach, and kale also provide substantial plant protein in our diets. Research has shown that plant protein is by far healthier to our bodies than animal protein, which lacks fiber and has little nutrient benefit in our diets.

## Calcium

Is dairy essential for strong bones?  Scientific research has proven that dairy *may not* be so good for our bones and may in fact raise Insulin-like Growth Factor 1 (IGF-1).  IGF-1 may promote cancer cell tumor growth in estrogen type cancers such as prostate, breast, and colon cancers.

Calcium is a necessary essential nutrient our bodies need, but you can opt for better, healthier choices in obtaining enough calcium through a whole foods plant-based diet by consuming foods that are rich in natural calcium, such as almonds, bok choy, broccoli, dark leafy greens, and vegetables.  Tempeh (a fermented soy), tofu, and edamame (soy beans) are great additions to our diet for obtaining calcium; however, remember these are soy foods and need to have the non-GMO label.

## Fats

By now you know that saturated fat is unhealthy and is found in all animal based foods: meat, fish, dairy, and eggs and should be avoided if you want to achieve a healthier lifestyle.  Our bodies require some fats but in the form of monounsaturated fat.  Healthier options for this would be consuming plant fats found in avocados, nuts, seeds, and olives. We want to keep oils to a minimum as well, such as extra virgin olive oil, coconut oil, grapeseed oil, and corn oil.  Studies have shown that oils are processed and are not healthy as once believed and may cause long term arterial damage which can lead to heart disease.

# Considerations for a Plant-Based Lifestyle

## Good Carbs vs. Bad Carbs

Quality does matter when it comes to consuming the right carbohydrates as some carbohydrates are healthier than others and it's important to know the difference. Many are confused about carbohydrates and therefore limit the amount they consume for fear of raising blood sugar or causing weight gain. You often hear people say, day after day, how tired they are, not realizing it may be their no carb or low carb diet causing their fatigue.

Carbohydrates provide our bodies with glucose, which is converted to energy and used to support bodily functions and physical activity. So, when you hear people saying they are tired all the time it may be that they are not consuming enough **complex carbohydrates** in their diet.

Unhealthy carbohydrates are called **simple carbohydrates** and you want to stay clear of these as they may contribute to weight issues and can promote heart disease and diabetes. These foods include white bread, pastries, sodas, highly processed foods, refined foods, white sugar, and white rice.

Foods high in **complex carbohydrates** are a very important part of a healthy diet. Complex carbohydrates are minimally processed whole grains, vegetables, fruits, and beans. These carbohydrates deliver vitamins, minerals, and fiber and provide our bodies with phytonutrients and energy throughout the day.

Complex carbohydrates include starches and dietary fiber. There are two types of fiber: soluble fiber and insoluble fiber and our bodies need both. Soluble fiber when digested absorbs water and creates a gel-like consistency. Examples would be psyllium, lentils, peas, and other legumes. Even apples, strawberries, and citrus fruits are soluble fibers. Soluble fiber slows the digestive process and helps maximize nutrient absorption.

Insoluble fiber is indigestible. It is not broken down and absorbed as soluble fiber, but instead adds bulk to our stools and reduces the transit time through the intestines. Examples of soluble fiber are whole grains as well as vegetables such as carrots, potatoes, and cabbage. Pears and prunes also contain insoluble fiber. Why are these both important? Soluble fiber prevents spikes in blood glucose for those challenging diabetes and aids in lowering cholesterol levels for the prevention of heart disease. Insoluble fiber will help to counteract constipation and diverticulosis. Studies have also shown that insoluble fiber can inhibit certain cancers such as colon cancer, which, according to the National Cancer Institute, is the second leading cause of cancer-related deaths.

Whole-grain foods are not only credited with adding high fiber in our diets but will boost your energy throughout the day. You will feel fuller longer, leaving you less hungry in between meals, which is a good thing.

Starchy foods are also important in a plant-based diet and include peas, corn, potatoes, beans, pasta, rice, and grains. Starchy foods are a main source of carbohydrates and play an important role in a healthy diet by providing our bodies with energy, fiber, and a wide range of nutrients. The potato, for instance, is considered a starchy food even though it is classified as a vegetable. Potatoes are not only a good source of energy and fiber but also B vitamins and potassium. Most people may think they are fattening, but this is only true with added ingredients like butter, cream sauces, and cheese.

Dairy-free and egg-free bread can be a challenge, but you can usually find them at your health food market or stores such as Whole Foods Market. Look for organic non-GMO tortilla wraps, oat, wheat, and multi-grain pita bread, 100% whole grain bread, sourdough, pumpernickel, and rye. If you have been diagnosed with diabetes, pumpernickel and rye bread are better choices for keeping blood sugar levels stable. If you're following a gluten-free diet along with your plant-based diet, be sure to read ingredient labels on gluten-free bread as many contain eggs.

Reading ingredient labels is a must when it comes to whole grain breads, tortillas and pita breads, as many contain hidden ingredients such as dairy, egg wash, high fructose corn syrup, and hydrogenated oils. Look for organic breads and wraps, which will avoid unhealthy ingredients.

## Snacks & Portion Control

Be careful and limit snacks available in stores. Even though they might be vegan you don't want these to substitute for healthier options such as whole grains, beans, vegetables, leafy greens, fruits, nuts, and seeds. Supermarket snacks, even though they may be vegan, are *empty calories with little nutrition.*

Portion control is a standard theme for most diets you see today. To be successful on a plant-based diet one needs to realize that eating a plant-based diet of vegetables, fruits, and leafy greens contains fewer calories but more nutrients and fiber than animal-based foods, which leave you with that "empty" feeling that encourages you to eat more calories. Plant foods are nutrient-dense foods that will help to maintain, satisfy your hunger, and improve your overall health and well-being.

## Viewpoint on Soy and Soy Products

There appears to be a lot of misconceptions and confusion on the issue of soy. You have heard me say over and over again that soy must be non-GMO. Genetically modified soy can cause adverse reactions such as allergies or other complications.

Most processed foods contain soy oils and corn oils. These soy and corn oils are GMO unless the product is labeled clearly that it is non-GMO or GMO-free. Non-GMO soy in the form of tofu, tempeh, soy milk, edamame (whole soybeans) and miso (fermented soy paste) are on the other hand healthy in moderation and cancer preventive.

A report on soy and health from the Physicians Committee for Responsible Medicine points out that soy products that are minimally processed are healthier soy options. Studies show that women who include soy products in their diet are less likely to develop breast cancer, compared with other women who consume no soy products. In fact, the study showed that women who consumed an average of one cup of soy milk or about one-half cup of tofu daily have about a 30% lower risk of developing breast cancer compared to those who ate *no* soy products. They noted, to be effective, the soy consumption may have to occur early in life, as breast tissue is formed during adolescence.

The *Woman's Healthy Eating and Living Study* showed that women who already have been diagnosed with breast cancer gain a major advantage by adding soy products into their diets and found that it may cut their risk of cancer recurrence or mortality in half. Further studies by the Journal of the American Medical Association reported results based on 5,042 women previously diagnosed with breast cancer who were participating in the Shanghai Breast Cancer Survival Study. Over a four-year period, women who consumed soy products, such as soy milk, tofu, or edamame had a 32% lower risk of recurrence and a 29% decreased risk of death, compared with women who consumed little or no soy. Continued research from Kaiser Permanente suggested much the same results and women who avoid soy products get no advantage at all.

Soy products have also been shown to have no adverse effects on men and may help prevent cancer in men. A study meta-analysis published in *Fertility and Sterility*, was based on more than 50 treatment groups, showed that neither soy products nor isoflavone supplements from soy affect testosterone levels in men. The American Journal of Clinical Nutrition showed that increased intake of soy resulted in a 26% reduction in prostate cancer risk and found a 30% risk reduction with non-fermented soy products such as soy milk and tofu.

Other studies have shown soy products may reduce the risk of fibroid tumors. Clinical studies in thyroid health show that soy products do not cause hypothyroidism; however, soy isoflavones may take up some of the iodine that the body would normally use to make thyroid hormones, thus adding iodine to their diet may be all that is needed. People with thyroid issues need to speak to their doctors as medications may need to be adjusted.

In summary, evidence to date indicates that soy products may reduce the risk of breast and prostate cancers. They do not appear to have adverse effects on the thyroid gland but may reduce the absorption of thyroid medications. The benefits of soy products appear to relate to traditional minimally processed soy, not to concentrated soy proteins.

# Special Dietary Considerations

## Gluten Free

Gluten free is now the growing rage sweeping across the map. Is gluten bad for us? The answer is only if you are gluten intolerant with celiac disease. Others find they may have a sensitivity, but the question is: it a wheat allergy or gluten that causes the sensitivity? Today we are now finding out that much of our wheat may be contaminated with glyphosate, a highly toxic herbicide that is sprayed on crops just before harvest and is believed to cause adverse side effects in our health.

Gluten-free products are a multimillion dollar business and tend to be very expensive. These are great products for those who cannot tolerate consuming gluten; however, in most cases this turns out to be a waste of money. Research has shown that most consumers derive no significant benefit from eating these products and perhaps is really a placebo affect one maybe experiencing. There are tests available to determine for sure if you are gluten or wheat intolerant.

Some people may see going gluten-free as just giving up traditional bread, pizza, pasta, and beer, when actually it's much more than that, especially if you have celiac disease. It may be in your sauces or hidden in products listed as natural flavorings. It may lurk in your shampoo, toothpaste, soap, cosmetics, medicines, and supplements making a gluten-free diet very challenging to contend with.

There are certain nutritional deficiencies that could be experienced with a gluten-free diet. Gluten-free foods are typically not fortified with vitamins. You may want to add a multivitamin to your day to counteract any deficiencies you may encounter. Another issue is dietary fiber that may be lacking in a gluten-free (GF) diet, which is important for our bowels to work properly. If you are following a GF diet you will want to add GF whole grains, such as brown rice, quinoa, millet, and polenta, along with fruits and vegetables. Most Americans. gluten-free or not, are deficient in fiber.

## Vegan Diet for Mothers, Mothers-to-Be and Children

Dr. Benjamin Spock wrote in his last revised edition, before he passed away in his 90's, that all children should be vegan. You may want to purchase this book for information that may be helpful choosing the correct nutrients for your child on a plant-based diet as their requirements for nutrients will be different than for an adult. If you are an expectant mother, you can be on a plant based diet as long as you are getting the correct number of nutrients needed for you and your unborn child.

I stress that it is important for mothers who are pregnant and for mothers who wish to change their infant and toddler's diets to plant-based that they speak with their doctor and a qualified licensed nutritionist who understands plant-based nutrition to be assured you and your child are getting the proper nutrients each and every day.

# Restocking your Refrigerator/Freezer and Pantry

You are now familiar with foods that may cause harm to your health and you have learned the importance of reading ingredient labels before purchasing products. You now know the concerns about genetically modified foods and where we obtain all of our nutrients on a plant-based diet. Now it's time to replace all the unhealthy foods with healthier options.

Many foods you may have already discarded, placed on a different shelf, or given away can be easily replaced with healthier ingredients. Here is a list of new healthier food choices for restocking your refrigerator, freezer, and pantry. Make time for your grocery shopping as reading ingredient labels will become a priority so unhealthy food items won't creep back into your pantry.

## Refrigerated Foods

Popular brand names for vegan products found in many grocery or health food stores are Daiya, Field Roast, Gardein, So Delicious, Silk, Tofurky, Lightlife, Just Mayo, Follow Your Heart, Earth Balance or Smart Balance. Remember, every state seems to carry different brand names. Most of the brands mentioned above can be found in most states.

It is important to point out that these store-bought food products replace animal proteins with plant proteins but they are still processed foods and should only be used in moderation to help you transition to a plant-based diet. We don't want these food items to replace whole foods such as beans/legumes, whole grains, vegetables, greens, fruits, nuts, and seeds. Non-GMO tofu, tempeh and homemade seitan (recipe available on Bob's Red Mill Vital Wheat Gluten packaging) are less processed meat alternative options.

- Dairy Free Milk- Soy Milk, Almond Milk, Rice Milk, Coconut Milk.
- Dairy and Egg Free Mayonnaise- Just Mayo, Follow Your Heart, Hellman's vegan.
- Non-Dairy Yogurt- Silk, So Delicious, Daiya Greek Yogurt. (look for diary free vegan)
- Egg Replacers - (flax meal, Ener-G Egg Replacer, Follow Your Heart VeganEgg).
- Non-Dairy Cheese products- Daiya Cheese, Follow Your Heart and Field Roast Cao Cheese. Be careful as some non-dairy cheese may read *lactose free* but still contain the dairy protein, casein. *Casein is, considered by many, a dangerous animal protein that has been found to cause tumor cell growth in laboratory studies. Avoid any non-dairy cheese with casein.*
- Vegan Parmesan Cheese.
- Vegan Cream Cheese (no casein).
- Vegan Sour Cream (no casein).
- Non-Dairy Creamers- Silk and So Delicious (no casein).
- Vegan Butter- Earth Balance or Smart Balance.
- Soy, Rice or Coconut whip cream- So Delicious makes a coconut cool whip non-dairy alternative and you can find Soyatoo soy or rice whip cream in a can at whole foods market in the refrigerated section of your store or health food market.
- Hummus and Guacamole.
- Tofu (non-GMO)- Vacuum sealed extra firm for use in entrees or firm and soft for desserts and sauces. *Silken* Tofu comes in a box and is not refrigerated. Soft and firm and extra-firm *silken* tofu are often used in recipes as an egg replacer, in desserts, and cream sauces. Cookbooks and online recipes will usually say whether the recipes call for

silken tofu or vacuum sealed tofu and whether to use extra-firm, firm, or soft.

## Fruits, Berries, Citrus, & Melons

- Fresh & Frozen Fruits- Apples, bananas, peaches, apricots, nectarines, plums, figs, pears, avocados.
- Fresh & Frozen Berries- Strawberries, blackberries, blueberries, raspberries.
- Citrus - Oranges, grapefruit (note some medications interact with grapefruit).
- Lemons and limes.
- Melons- Cantaloupe, honey dew, and watermelon.
- Tropical - Mango, papaya, pineapple, kiwi, jicama, fresh coconut.

## Fresh Vegetables and Greens

- Vegetables- Sweet peppers, green peppers, zucchini, yellow squash, cucumbers, tomatoes, winter squash, onions (red, yellow, sweet, green, leeks, shallots), ginger, garlic cloves, green beans, asparagus, carrots, radishes, Brussels sprouts, broccoli, cauliflower, cabbage, bean sprouts, fennel, potatoes (all varieties, however, more nutrients in sweet potatoes and try purple potatoes).
- Leafy Greens – Bok choy, kale, Swiss chard, dandelion, collard, romaine, butter leaf, spinach, arugula and red leaf lettuce. Avoid head lettuce (iceberg), which has very little nutritional value.

## Freezer Foods

- Meat Substitutes- Gardein, Beyond Meat, Tofurkey, Field Roast, Lightlife and Butler Soy Curls. Be sure they are organic and non-GMO.
- Tempeh (non-GMO)- Lightlife is my favorite brand.

- West Soy Seitan- Found in most health foods stores or at Whole Foods Market.
- Vacuum Sealed Tofu can be frozen or refrigerated.
- Organic frozen vegetables.
- Organic frozen potatoes- Alexia sweet potato fries, hash browns, crinkles, and wedges.
- Whole Grain Waffles.
- Whole Grain Pancakes.
- Non-Dairy Ice Cream (as a special treat now and then).
- Non-Dairy Ice Treats (as a special treat now and then).
- Non-Dairy Sorbets (as a special treat now and then).
- Non-Dairy Cheesecake – Daiya cheesecake. Available New York style, Strawberry, Key Lime and Chocolate.
- Non-Dairy pie crust (Wholly Wholesome offers organic whole grain and gluten free options.
- Organic Graham Cracker Pie Shell from Arrow Head Mills.

## Pantry Staples

- Tomatoes- Stewed, diced, fire roasted, crushed, tomato paste, and tomato sauce.
- Spaghetti and Marinara sauces. Organic if possible to avoid high fructose corn syrup.
- Artichoke Hearts
- Capers
- Roasted Red Peppers
- Olive Tapenade
- Olives- canned, bottled or fresh
- Pickles
- Sauerkraut
- Vegan Salad Dressings
- Organic Ketchup/Mustard/Hot Sauces

- Organic marinade sauces
- Organic Soy Sauce or Bragg's Liquid Aminos gluten-free soy alternative.
- Vegan Worcestershire Sauce
- Organic canned or dried Beans- Red, White, Black, Kidney, Black-Eyed Peas, Pinto.
- Whole Grain Pasta or Gluten-Free pasta.
- Whole Grain Organic non-GMO crackers/Chips.
- Whole Grains- Quinoa, brown rice (long and short grain), black rice, wild rice, buckwheat, polenta, millet, wheatberries, farro, organic freekeh (green wheat). Avoid white rice, which raises our blood sugar levels.

## Essential Products for Plant-Based Recipes

**Nutritional Yeast-** (not brewer's yeast, there is a difference) Nutritional yeast is a deactivated yeast, often a strain of *Saccharomyces cerevisiae*, which is sold commercially as a food product and is usually fortified with B-12. It is sold in the form of flakes or as a yellow powder. Nutritional yeast is very cheesy tasting and can be used on Italian dishes in place of Parmesan cheese. It is also very tasty when sprinkled on popcorn. We recommend Nutritional yeast products from *Bragg's* or *Bob's Red Mill*. You can order *Now* brand at iHerb.com which is pharmaceutical grade and assures you are getting all the necessary B vitamins in your diet.

**Vegetable Broth-** Buy organic. To make your own homemade vegetable broth, a nice blend of carrots, onions, celery, parsley (fresh), fresh thyme (or any other fresh herbs) and whole peppercorns makes a lovely broth. You can also add parsnips, mushrooms, fennel, tomatoes or leeks. Bring to a boil and then simmer for about one hour or so. Then strain into a mason jar. Storing food in glass jars and containers are a better option. If using plastic be sure they are BPA-free. Vegetable broth can be frozen.

Note: one thing I always do when using vegetable broth whether store bought or homemade in a recipe is to add 1 tablespoon of soy sauce or Bragg's Liquid Aminos (Gluten-Free soy alternative) to my broth. If a recipe calls for 6 cups of broth add 1 tablespoon of soy sauce to the pot. It will enrich your broth with a wonderful savory flavor.

**No-Chicken Broth** –*Imagine Foods* brand "no-chicken broth" (comes in a box), which is also great to have on hand when a recipe may call for chicken broth.

**Bouillon** – *Better than Bouillon* makes a wonderful broth that comes as no chicken, no beef, vegetable, and mushroom. It is a paste in a glass jar and you just add 1 teaspoon of the paste for each cup of water.

**Sauces** – There are several organic sauces on the market for stir-frying or for marinating. These include: teriyaki sauce, orange sauce, hoisin sauce, peanut sauce, Thai sauces, curry, some steak sauces, and vegan Worcestershire sauce. Many varieties of hot sauces are great for spicing up dishes and include: Asian chili paste, Sriracha sauce or our favorite, *Valentina Salsa Picante* Mexican hot sauce.

**Himalayan Black Salt**- (actually pink in color) This is not to be confused with Himalayan sea salt. Himalayan black salt (also known as Kala Namak) has a high sulfur content that provides a pungent aroma resembling egg. It is often used in recipes like tofu scramble or chickpea omelets to give the recipe an egg flavor. You will find this black salt at your local Indian markets or you can order though *Amazon*.

***Ditch the table salt,*** which is highly processed and has no nutritional value and switch to sea salt, such as Himalayan Pink Salt or Celtic Sea Salt, which are better options. These salts are unprocessed, retaining many minerals you may be lacking from your diet.

If you are on a salt-free diet you can use many of the *No-Salt* seasonings on the market today.

You are going to go through a learning process when it comes to vegan ingredients and only then will you begin to understand why they are used to create certain flavors. Don't be afraid to try an ingredient because it is foreign in name as you may be missing out on some of the best flavors ever!

## Spices and Herbs (dried and fresh)

- **Spices:** turmeric, cumin, fennel, cardamom, mustard powder, poultry seasoning, coriander, five spice (Asian), garam masala & curry powder (Indian), nutmeg, cloves, cinnamon, paprika (sweet and smoked), ginger powder.

- **Herbs:** rosemary, basil, sage, thyme, oregano, parsley, savory, herbs de Provence, Italian seasoning, dill weed, marjoram, salt free *Mrs. Dash*, sea salt, black pepper, red pepper flakes, onion powder and garlic powder.

*See More in the Chapter on Spices and Herbs.*

# Our Four New Food Groups

## Designing a Powerful Plate

Let's look at our dinner plate and divide it into quarters to show how a plant-based diet works.

One section will now be filled with **vegetables** that also includes starchy vegetables. The second section will be filled with **whole grains**. The third section will be our **protein** choice and the fourth section **fruit**. You can eat these foods individually or combine them into a recipe of your choosing.

1. Vegetables: choose a variety of different vegetables and greens. Starchy vegetables include potatoes, parsnips, corn, squash (both summer and winter varieties), plantains, and green peas. Choosing a variety of vegetables and not concentrating on just one insures we are consuming all the necessary nutrients needed for our health.

2. Whole grains: include bread, brown rice, quinoa, pasta, hot or cold cereal, corn, millet, barley, bulgur, buckwheat, groats, and tortillas. Whole grains are rich in fiber and other complex carbohydrates and provide us with protein, B vitamins and zinc.

3. We are now replacing *animal* protein with *plant* protein such as beans and legumes, nuts and seeds, tofu, tempeh and seitan. There are many vegan meatless analogues available at most supermarkets today, such as meatless meatballs, ground crumbles, chicken strips, and beefless tips that can help you transition away from animal protein and replace your meals with protein from plant sources.

4. Fruit is our go-to dessert or sweet treat. Most Americans are deficient when it comes to eating fruit every day. Choose whole fruit over fruit juices, which do not contain the fiber that whole fruits offer.

## Preparing Your Power Plate

Now that you've got a glimpse of what foods you can enjoy with a plant-based diet, the real trick is motivating ourselves into our kitchens, cooking and preparing healthy meals rather than eating out at fast food restaurants or placing a frozen dinner into our microwave ovens. This will be challenge at first, however, the more you practice real cooking the better you become.

You will soon realize that dicing and slicing vegetables isn't difficult and the more you do it the easier and quicker it becomes as you find your own shortcuts that work for you and your family. A huge incentive, by the way, is how much money you will be saving by not eating out at restaurants on a daily basis!

It's a great time to involve everyone in the kitchen to learn about food and how it is prepared. You might be surprised how many children (and adults) have no clue what certain vegetables and fruit are, where they come from, or how they are grown. If these foods are never being served in your home, then you can't expect children to know that French fries and ketchup is not a salad. You get my point! Children love to be in the kitchen, they love helping mom or dad, and surprisingly they love to eat what they prepare. They may even try that broccoli now!

Our nation has a growing problem called obesity that is spinning out of control and not just in adults. Unfortunately, our children are being diagnosed with type 2 diabetes and heart disease before even reaching adulthood, and are being prescribed lifelong medications for conditions that are preventable with diet change. If this trend continues this will be the first generation of children who die before their parents. We are a nation where children are growing up thinking fast food is food, restaurants our kitchen, and microwaves our oven. Many are going off to college and have no clue how to cook a nutritious meal. This should be a wakeup call for all parents! If we as adults can't change, then how can we expect our children not to want these same foods that make us sick?

Let's be blunt here: It's easier to make time for all our activities and driving to a fast food restaurant (or any restaurant for that matter), than making time in our day to allow 30 minutes to cook a nutritious meal for your family and maybe just maybe prevent an early onset disease that could affect a loved one's life.

# Changes You Can Expect on a Whole Foods Plant-Based Diet

Thomas Alva Edison believed *"The doctor of the future will give no medicine, but will instruct his patient in the care of the human frame in diet and in the cause and prevention of disease."*

Unfortunately, today doctors treat our symptoms (and that is what they are trained to do), but we need to look at the *cause* of the disease. Symptoms are masked with prescription drugs and come with side effects that can make you sicker. Did you know that side effects from pharmaceutical drugs is the third leading killer of people today? It's time to concentrate on the *cause* of our illness or disease and not mask it with a temporary band aid and suffer the possible side effects from medications which, in many cases, are worse than the original illness being treated and land many in the hospital with life-threating reactions.

A whole foods plant-based diet is powerful and one can expect to see changes in their bodies, not in years, but in *weeks* or *months*. Many will discover that constipation will disappear (the average American is deficient in fiber) and bowel movement will be easier, more frequent, and will continually remove toxins from our bodies. You may notice a significant drop in cholesterol and blood sugar return to normal range. A diet rich in plant foods are health-enhancing, offering antioxidants that fight free radicals that can damage our cells. Many who follow a plant-based diet notice a surge in energy levels, which keeps us moving when age tries to slow us down. A whole foods plant-based diet helps us to remove unwanted pounds easily if we need to lose weight and maintain our weight efficiently and safely as it is not an on-again/off-again diet, but a lifestyle change.

## Internal Changes

At the moment, we feel pretty good and we may look pretty healthy, but are we *really* healthy?  We hear all the time about a sports figure or a marathon runner who suddenly dies while performing.  We don't think about diet effecting internal changes such as arterial damage caused by unhealthy foods; after all, we can't see inside our bodies, so why worry about it?

A whole foods plant-based diet works behind the scenes by clearing our blood vessels and providing more oxygen into our bodies.  It builds a strong immune system and helps prevent cancer, type 2 diabetes and heart disease.  Many experience lower blood pressure and hormones become balanced. You may experience fewer colds and infections and fewer sick days.  Our bones become stronger and you feel less fatigue throughout the day.  Best of all, you are rewarded with good health and longevity as your healthy food choices now aid your body to become disease resistant as your immune system begins operating at optimum levels.

## Addressing the Cause, Not the Symptom

Remember, most doctors treat *symptoms* and plant-based nutrition impacts *causes*.

Don't get me wrong here: doctors are great and we need them!  Combining medicine *with* nutrition however, will support healing and bring about better results in our health and wellness.

We have been abusing our bodies for many years now, not only with food but the overuse of prescription and over the counter drugs.  When we start a healthy diet, our immune system kicks in, and we may experience what is known as "detox symptoms" for a few days.  Food can be an addiction for many and detox symptoms may often be experienced as a form of withdrawal. Some symptoms you might experience may be:

- Joint or muscle pain
- Diarrhea
- Fatigue
- Headache
- Cold or flu-like symptoms
- Strong emotions

These *flu-like* symptoms will disappear in a few days and may not happen to everyone. If major symptoms happen, please check with your doctor as something else maybe going on.

Unfortunately, we live in a toxic world whether it's the environment, foods we consume, or the products we use to clean our home or the water we bathe in. We will always have toxins to fight off, but keeping our immune system working at top performance will help us fight these toxins, which is what our immune system is designed to do.

The next time you go shopping observe what customers are buying. Do you see fresh vegetables, greens, whole grains, and fresh fruit? Most carts are just the opposite: overloaded with boxes of highly processed foods, microwave dinners, diet drinks, candy, and desserts. If you shop at a wholesale membership or other big-box store, you will most often see grocery carts are overflowing with even larger cases and quantities of highly processed foods, sodas, desserts, and pounds of meat, fish, dairy, and eggs. This represents our Standard American Diet and hence the nickname SAD.

Laboratory studies have now shown that eating large amounts of animal protein has adverse effects on our health. The SAD diet will gradually and eventually impact your body and be reflected in signs of obesity, heart disease, type 2 diabetes and cancer. It's only a matter of time!

Unfortunately, there is no magic pill or we would all be taking it! The magic begins when we take responsibility for our own health and family wellness. The magic begins when you see results in just a few weeks or months what a plant-based diet can do. Consuming *whole* foods, not *fake* foods, is real magic!

## Other Challenges

It's natural for people to concentrate at first on all of the foods they can't eat when making a diet change. Push those thoughts aside and make a list of all the healthy food choices you *can* eat. As you experiment in the kitchen you will understand more and see that your favorite meals can be made plant-based with a few minor substitutions and without the use of meat, fish, dairy, or eggs. Your meals will still look, smell, and taste wonderful!

There will be other challenges you will encounter, for instance, holiday time. Tradition is a huge turkey, ham, or roast on our dining room tables for the holidays; after all, it is how we were raised and family traditions are a hard thing to break as they are connected to so many memories. You can still enjoy all of your holidays with the same tantalizing tastes, smells, and colors, but in a much healthier way. There are many meat alternative "roasts" that are plant-based and delicious. There are many plant-based vegan cookbooks and online holiday recipes to help you make this transition easy; in fact, you will enjoy your holidays even more knowing the meal is healthier and understanding that holiday time is really a time of being together with the people you love. If you are attending a holiday meal at a friend's or other family member's house ask the host if you could bring a few plant-based dishes for everyone to enjoy, relieving the host of worrying what to fix for their vegan guest. High fat meals at holiday time land many in the hospital with their first heart attack.

Another challenge is eating out. I see more and more restaurants adding vegan meals to their menus, but for many restaurants you just need to ask if the chef can prepare a vegan meal. When attending a night out with your friends at a restaurant ask first where they will be eating and call ahead or go online and check out their menu. Many people acquiesce or "cheat" when eating out. It's certainly tempting to see everything that is on a menu and in some cases, may find nothing you can eat. Should that occur, look at the vegetable side dishes and salads. Ask if they are cooked or prepared with butter or added cheese. Ask if there is dairy or eggs in their pasta or breads. Baked potatoes are usually found on most menus; ask if the chef can top it with fresh steamed veggies and order a side of extra virgin olive oil to drizzle on top.

Most restaurants employ good chefs who should be able to fix something nice for you and if he or she can't, well maybe no one should be eating there in the first place! Keep in mind when eating out all the time that restaurants are not geared toward health; they don't worry if you are obese, diabetic, or have cancer or heart disease. They are there to serve you food and not necessarily concerned whether the dish is high in fat, sugar, cholesterol, or sodium.

Grocery shopping is also a challenge. We all have good intentions when it comes to shopping and buying whole foods. We enter the store and fill our carts with fresh vegetables and fruits and admire their colors and are excited to get home and place them neatly in the refrigerator while still admiring their beauty. But there they sit day after day. It's now a week and they are going bad. So, what happened? You forgot to eat them and more than likely, because you didn't know how to prepare them. This becomes a waste of money and discourages many from eating a healthy diet.

The easy recipes offered at the end of this book will help you learn to create recipes using vegetables, greens, fruits and whole grains that your entire family will love. One thing I have learned transitioning from an animal-based diet to a plant-based diet is to create dishes that your family is already familiar with and enjoy, such as spaghetti and "meat" balls or vegetable lasagna. All types of cuisine are possible and can be made vegan, such as Mexican dishes, Italian dishes, Mediterranean dishes, Indian dishes, tropical dishes, and Asian Dishes. Let your imagination go wild!

# Buying Greens and Vegetables in the Produce Aisle

### Does every fruit and vegetable need to be organic?

This choice is up to each person's financial capabilities and preferences. I will be the first to say I don't always buy organic. I do when possible and if not, I do buy from our local farmer's market to avoid GMOs. I carry a list in my wallet called the *"Dirty Dozen* and *Clean 15"*. This list shows which fruits and vegetables need to be organic and which ones you can buy conventionally or locally grown using fewer pesticides. If you happen to be in a store with no organic produce, choose vegetables that are greenhouse grown as they will usually have fewer pesticides.

## *Dirty* Dozen

- Apples
- Celery
- Strawberries
- Peaches
- Spinach
- Nectarines
- Grapes – imported
- Sweet Bell Peppers
- Potatoes
- Blueberries – domestic
- Lettuce
- Kale/Collard Greens

## *Clean 15*

- Onions
- Sweet Corn

- Pineapples
- Avocado
- Asparagus
- Sweet peas
- Mangoes
- Eggplant
- Cabbage
- Cantaloupe- domestic
- Kiwi
- Watermelon
- Sweet potatoes
- Grapefruit
- Mushrooms
- Tomatoes

Tip: When buying fruit, vegetables, and greens find the product code, which is the sticker on your produce. This sticker tells you a lot:

*5-Digit Code starting with 9 means Organic*
*4-Digit Code starting with 4 means Conventional*
*5-Digit Code starting with 8 means GMO*

The produce aisle can be daunting if you are one who spends little time there; however, this section of the grocery store is going to become your friend and new medicine cabinet. Here you will find all the nutrients, fiber, and antioxidants our bodies crave. In this section, you will go through many of the common produce items used in many vegan plant-based recipes. Do you need them all at once? Certainly not! Each week find a new vegetable or green that you have never tried before and as you continue to do this, you will soon find you are consuming the rainbow!

Did you know that almost all vegetables contain protein? This may surprise many. Peas, spinach, kale, broccoli, sprouts, mushrooms, Brussels sprouts, artichokes, asparagus, and corn are high protein vegetables!

## How to Prepare, Cook, and Store Your Greens

How important is it to eat your greens? Very important! When you think one bowl of greens is sufficient then triple that bowl! I do hope you will give them a try as it is one of the healthiest foods for your body.

*Do check with your doctor if you are taking certain heart medications such as blood thinners. Your doctor may have to adjust your dosage differently if you are consuming leafy green vegetables on a regular basis.*

## *Kale*

Kale is known for its lowering of cholesterol as well lowering our risk of certain types of cancer that include bladder, breast, colon, ovary, and prostate. Isothiocyanates or ITCs made from glucosinolates in kale play the primary role of cancer prevention. Kale helps our bodies to detoxify at a genetic level. The flavonoids in kale offer protection with its high antioxidant and anti-inflammatory benefits. Its health benefits are the same as those in cruciferous vegetables which are also cancer protective.

Be sure to pick kale that is green with no yellow spots or wilted leaves or tiny holes. Smaller size leaves will be more tender and milder in flavor. Kale is now available year-round with its peak season in winter through spring. It is very easy to grow in your garden from seed. Look for organic seeds.

Kale likes a cool environment and will stay fresh in your refrigerator for about five days sealed in a plastic bag with the air taken out. Longer storage makes the leaves more bitter so best to use your kale within the five days and then buy more. Only wash your kale when ready to use as moisture will promote spoilage.

The first step is to clean each leaf under cold running water. I like to remove the center stem which can be tough to eat then cut or tear the leaf into ¼-inch pieces. Using a large pan such as a wok works great or a 12-inch pan will hold your greens. Don't be alarmed as to how much it appears to be in your pan; as you begin to steam them in a little water they will begin to wilt. I like to add a touch of olive oil, a squeeze of lemon juice, and minced garlic to the pan. You may want to put a lid on for a few minutes to help them steam. Steaming enhances their healthy benefit.

## *Swiss Chard*

Swiss chard is another green providing our bodies with phytonutrients that contain several antioxidants and also aids in keeping blood sugar levels balanced. You will find some Swiss chard with red stems. The reddish-purple veins and stems provide our bodies with anti-inflammatory properties and detoxification support. Swiss chard also comes with white stems. White stems are more tender and can be eaten, whereas red stems tend to be tougher. If buying with red stems be sure to de-stem your Swiss chard. If buying white stem, you can eat those along with the leaves.

When buying Swiss chard look for bright green leaves that are not yellowed or browned and the stalks that are firm and without blemish.

To store Swiss chard, place unwashed in a plastic bag and take out the air. It will remain fresh in your refrigerator for five days. Swiss chard can also be blanched and frozen for future use.

First step is to wash each leaf under cold water. Stack each leaf on top of each other and then then begin to chop down to the stem. If your stem is white, continue to chop. If your stem is red, stop chopping as this stem will be very tough to eat.

Swiss chard is best boiled which helps to release its acidic components and will make it sweeter in taste. Do not drink the water from the pot after boiling as it will be very acidic. Use a large soup pot with water and bring to a boil add your white stems first (no red stems) and boil for about 2 minutes. Then add your leaves and boil for about 3 minutes. Be sure to time the 3 minutes as you don't want to overcook them. Pour your water and greens into a strainer and press out the water being careful not to burn yourself. Add your favorite dressing or add a drizzle of red wine vinegar.

## Collard Greens

Collard greens are beneficial for lowering cholesterol and also cancer prevention by supporting our detox and anti-inflammatory responses.

When buying collard greens, look for firm leaves that are not wilted or show signs of yellowing or browning. Smaller leaves will be more tender in texture and flavor. Once again store in your refrigerator in a plastic bag with the air taken out. If the leaves are too large, then de-stem them and cut the leaves to fit into a plastic bag. You may want to leave some with the stem on if you will be using them for vegetable wraps. Collard greens will stay fresh for 3-5 days in cool storage.

First begin by rinsing collard leaves under cold water. If I am using collard greens for a certain dish I am making such as soups and stews I like to de-stem the collards and place each leaf on top of the other and roll up. Next *chiffonade* into strips and add to your soup or stew at the very end of cooking, just until they wilt and are tender. If I am using my collards as a side dish I like to steam my collard greens in a wok or 12-inch pan with a little olive oil, garlic, and lemon juice. To serve, add your favorite dressing or red wine vinegar. You can also leave the stem on your collard greens and shave the stem thinly and boil for only 3 minutes (use a timer). Use the same as you would use cabbage leaves for roll ups with a rice and bean mixture inside and top with diced canned fire-roasted tomatoes.

## Dandelion Greens

Dandelion greens belong to the sunflower family. Most people would probably pass them buy at the supermarket not realizing all the health benefits of adding these to your meals. They are loaded with vital nutrients and fiber that help with digestion, strengthening our bones, heart health and cancer prevention. Dandelion greens can be added to your salads or try adding them to your next soup or stew. I like to combine them with other greens but you can make a dandelion salad exclusively mixed with other veggies for a healthy nutritious meal.

To store your dandelion leaves do not wash but place in a plastic bag and squeeze out the air and store in your refrigerator. Only wash greens when you're ready to consume. If you prefer you can quickly blanch and plunge into cold water and place in a freezer bag or container in your freezer. Dandelion greens should last for 3-5 days in the refrigerator.

## Bok Choy

Bok choy falls in the cruciferous vegetable family. Nutritionally it is one of the highest ranked vegetables, providing our bodies with 21 nutrients including omega-

3s and over 70 antioxidants to protect our cells. This is one plant you will want to add to your plant-based diet on a regular basis. To store bok choy, place the entire head in a plastic bag and remove as much air as possible and store in your vegetable crisper drawer. Stored properly, bok choy can last up to one week. Remember to look for bok choy with fresh leaves that are not wilted, yellowed or brown. I prefer to buy baby bok choy as they are more tender then larger heads. I like to steam my bok choy just until tender. If using in a recipe such as stir fry or soups and stew, simply chop off the bottom, wash leaves in cold water, then chop into chunks and add to your stir fry, soup, or stew.

## Mustard Greens

Mustard greens are another green in the cruciferous plant family and one to add to your recipes for their health benefits. They are great addition to your diet for cardiovascular health, and they contain anti-inflammatory properties. Mustard greens tend to be on the spicy side like mustard. I tend to use these sparingly in a recipe, adding a few sprigs mixed with other greens, but some may like a spicier flavor and can add more. To store mustard greens, do not wash before placing them in a plastic bag. Squeeze out as much air as possible and wash when ready to consume. Mustard greens will stay fresh for about 4-5 days. Mustard greens are best sautéed in 5 tablespoons of vegetable broth or water for about 5 minutes. If you would like to eat a side dish of mustard greens serve with a healthy Mediterranean type salad dressing.

## Spinach

Spinach is rich in vitamins and minerals. Because of its phytonutrients spinach has anti-inflammatory and anti-cancer properties. You all remember "Popeye"! Spinach is high in vitamin C, A, and E, manganese, zinc and selenium, reducing oxidative stress throughout our bodies. It is a rich source of calcium and magnesium which helps to support our bone health.

To store spinach, place it unwashed inside a plastic bag and take out as much air as possible. Place in your refrigerator for up to five days. Look for spinach leaves and stems that are bright green and not pale or yellowed. Avoid those that look wilted or bruised. Signs of decaying are leaves that become slimy and it's time to discard.

To clean fresh spinach, you will want to soak them lightly in a bowl of cold water which will help to rinse off any dirt and debris, then do a second wash the same way. Do not leave the leaves in water as it will begin to leach out the nutrients. If you buy your spinach in pre-washed plastic containers simply rinse in a colander and shake to dry out or use a salad spinner to dry.

## Romaine Lettuce

Think of Romaine as the new "head lettuce"; one of the healthiest greens to add to your salads, loaded with vitamins and minerals. Want to keep your heart healthy? Throw away head (iceberg) lettuce, which has no nutritional value and replace with romaine in your next salad! To store keep in plastic bag with air pressed out and store in refrigerator. You can wash the leaves first but be sure to dry leaves well before storing in your refrigerator. I have wrapped a paper towel around washed leaves and placed in a plastic bag with air pressed out and it works well also.

## Turnip Greens

Turnip greens again are in the cruciferous plant family. They are high in calcium and phytonutrients called glucosinolates which are cancer-preventing. Look for turnip greens that are without blemishes, show crispness, and are deep green in color. Remove the greens from their roots and store them separately in a plastic bag unwashed, taking out as much air in the plastic bag as possible. Turnip greens will stay fresh for up to four days. To cook, steaming is the recommended process. Fill your steamer pot with water and place washed greens in steamer basket and steam for 5 minutes. Use a timer so as not to overcook. When finished, you can add red wine vinegar to your greens or your favorite vegan vinaigrette dressing.

## Beet Greens

As you shop for beets you will find they have their tops attached. Most often people cut the greens away from the beets and cook the beets discarding the greens; however, the greens contain many healthy nutrients. Since vegans do not consume dairy you are often asked where you get your calcium and magnesium. Greens are high in folic acid and a good source of lutein which is good for eye health and other chronic diseases such as diabetes, cardiovascular disease, and cancer. When choosing beet greens (attached to their beet root) choose smaller beets rather than large ones as they will be tender. Look for beet roots that are not cracked, soft, bruised, or very dry-looking or shriveled. Watch for scaly-looking beets as they will tend to be tougher. The leaves should not be wilted but crisp and fresh looking and bright green.

To store your beets do not wash but separate the leaves from the root and place in separate plastic bags and press out the air and store in your refrigerator. Wash when ready to consume. They will keep for approximately four days. To cook your beet greens, boil in a large pot of water, which helps to remove their acid content. First bring your water to a boil and then place your beet greens into the pot and time for one minute. Do not cover your pot. Strain your pot and press out remaining liquid in your greens and add your favorite vinaigrette or red wine vinegar for added flavor.

## *Arugula*

Arugula is from the brassica family of vegetables along with broccoli, cauliflower, and cabbage. It is high in fiber and antioxidants and rich in chlorophyll, which helps to prevent liver and DNA damage. Arugula is 90% water and is what is called a hydrating leafy green. Arugula contains vitamin K which is beneficial for bone health and this leafy green helps to reduce inflammation in the body. It is a good body detoxifier because of its antioxidant qualities and essential minerals. Arugula is also high in B vitamins and protects our brain from cognitive decline. It is low in calories and a perfect addition to your meals for weight loss and helps to block environmental contaminants you come into contact with daily.

Arugula leaves should be long, firm, and bright green. Larger leaves are more peppery than smaller leaves. Avoid leaves that are discolored or bruised or past their expiration date. Most of the time you will find arugula in the store in a plastic container and it is fine to keep in the container as is. If you are buying loose leaves, wrap the stems or roots in a moistened paper towel and place leaves in a plastic bag in the most humid area of your refrigerator. Most arugula packaged leaves have a two-week shelf life. If you purchase as a bunch, it has a two- to three-day shelf life. Arugula can tend to be gritty so be sure to rinse leaves thoroughly before consuming. Arugula is great to add to salads and also stirred into pasta dishes and on top of pizza. I have also used it in sandwich wraps and as a great topping on baked potatoes.

# Enjoy Your Greens

Greens are the crowning jewel of all good health. You can steam or sauté as a side dish. Large green leaves like collard, kale and Swiss chard make wonderful veggie wraps and can be used in place of bread for a lower caloric sandwich. More ways to enjoy your greens:

- Juice your greens, adding an apple and carrot in your juicer
- Make a smoothie with spinach, pineapple, blueberries, and coconut water
- Make a large salad mixed with several different greens and top with sprouts
- Add chopped greens to soups and stews
- Briefly wilt a handful of greens in your pasta dishes
- Make a Buddha bowl with brown rice, greens, vegetables, and hummus dressing
- Add greens to your stir fry

Dark leafy greens are a great source of nutrition. They contain vitamin K, and are rich in many of the B vitamins. They also contain an abundance of antioxidants that are cancer protective. Greens are high in fiber, iron, magnesium, potassium, and calcium.

Once a week experiment with a new green in your diet. Choose from one of the following:

- Arugula
- Romaine
- Spinach
- Baby Bok Choy
- Sprouts
- Collard Greens
- Swiss Chard
- Kale

- Dandelion
- Mustard Greens (quite spicy; use just a sprig added to other greens)
- Turnip Greens

# Choosing Vegetables

Choosing vegetables are next on our grocery list. I have found over the past several years that most recipes use many of the same vegetables. Most are very common, easy to find, and inexpensive to buy. Once again you don't have to buy them all at once, but having a few of each in your refrigerator will allow you to cook a meal in no time without having to run to the store at the last minute. Some people dislike the taste of vegetables; please give them a second chance. It is amazing how eating animal proteins tend to deaden our taste buds and once you switch to a plant-based diet, which cleanses our taste buds, vegetables taste incredibly good again!

Try different cooking methods. My favorite is steaming and roasting vegetables. Boiling vegetables tends to take out all the nutrients and leaves you with limp, colorless, and mostly tasteless veggies. Vegetables should be enjoyed a little crisp rather than limp.

## Common Vegetables

Key nutrients found in vegetables are calcium, fiber, folate, iron, magnesium, potassium, sodium, and vitamins A & C. Remember almost ALL vegetables contain protein; just some more than others.

**Tomatoes-** Include both cherry and Roma for variation in your dishes. Even though tomatoes are technically a fruit, most consider them a vegetable.

**Red, Orange, & Yellow Peppers-** These sometimes can be expensive. Look for the mini bag now sold in most grocery stores that include all three colors: red, yellow, and orange.

**Green Peppers-** large peppers are great for stuffing.

**Sweet Corn-** Remember corn can be a GMO. Organic sweet corn can be found fresh, canned, or frozen.

**Artichokes-** Fresh artichokes are delicious for serving on a plate. To use artichokes as an ingredient in your favorite recipe, look for artichoke hearts in a can or in a jar preferably. They come plain or marinated.

**Asparagus-** Delicious steamed and raw on salads.

**Cauliflower-** Some call it a new potato. You can mash, roast, and steam cauliflower. There are many recipes that use cauliflower in place of meat and incorporating delicious sauces can replace dishes commonly made with chicken. Instead of chicken wings, try cauliflower wings or Korean fried cauliflower or Kung Pao cauliflower.

**Broccoli-** Such a versatile vegetable that can be used in every dish whether it be soup or a stew, stir fry, or a salad and works wonders in casseroles.

**Green Beans-** Frozen or fresh all come in handy for adding to soups and stews or steamed just right with a little crunch.

**Snow peas-** Snow peas are delicious in a stir fry and other Asian dishes.

**Sugar Snaps-**Sweet and delicious

**Mixed Salad Greens-** Today you can find a variety of mixed greens on the supermarket shelves. Experiment with several to find your favorites.

**Potatoes (all)-** Try steaming your potatoes rather than boiling. Boiled potatoes tend to drink up water and can make them soggy. Steaming prevents this. When baking potatoes, try something different by adding a combination of beans, vegetables, greens, and a drizzle of hot sauce or hummus dressing on your next baked potato.

**Onions-** Experiment using different varieties for your dishes: white, yellow, sweet Vidalia, red, green, scallions, and leeks. Onions have special compounds that fight free radicals in our bodies.

**Celery-** Contains a high percentage of water and has special compound that acts as a diuretic. It is both an antioxidant and anti-inflammatory and contains beneficial enzymes needed for our bodies. It is an anti-hypertensive vegetable that protects our cardiovascular system.

**Fresh Ginger-** Great for stir-fries and adding to Asian recipes.

**Garlic-** A wonderful addition to all dishes for adding flavor and fighting free radicals in our bodies. One can never have too much garlic in their diet.

**Fennel-** This an interesting vegetable. If you were to eat it raw it imparts a licorice flavor, but when steamed and added to your soups, stews, and other cuisine, it imparts a very delicate and outstanding flavor addition to your meals.

**Beets-** Pickled beets or fresh beets added to a salad is divine. You won't be disappointed!

**Cabbage-** Red (preferable, higher in antioxidants) and green. Add cabbage to soups, stews, and stir fry. Shredded raw cabbage added to your salad kicks it up a notch with that added crunch.

**Jicama-** This root vegetable was first grown in South and Central America. It is sweet tasting and crunchy; a cross between a potato and an apple, but does not have an edible skin. Try Jicama on your next salad which gives a sweet fresh taste and crunch to each bite.

Don't forget frozen vegetables! They are always good to have on hand when fresh are not available or you have no time to shop. Organic sweet corn, mixed vegetables, edamame (soy beans), peas, carrots, broccoli.

## Winter and Summer Squash

**Zucchini (summer squash)-** Can be eaten raw, spiralized into noodles or added to soups and stir fry (A spiralizer is a gadget that makes certain vegetables like zucchini, potatoes and yellow squash into noodles).

**Yellow Squash (summer squash)-** Can be eaten raw, spiralized into noodles, or added to soups and stir fry

**Butternut Squash (winter squash)-** Has a sweet and creamy orange flesh. It can be baked, mashed, pureed, steamed, simmered, or stuffed, and many times it is used in recipes as a substitute for sweet potatoes.

**Acorn Squash (winter squash)-** Can be stuffed or added to soups and stews.

**Spaghetti Squash (winter squash)-** Spaghetti squash gets its name as the flesh of the squash is spaghetti-like after baking. The more yellow a spaghetti squash is on the outside the better it is on the inside and larger ones are more flavorsome then smaller ones. Using a fork and scraping the inside of the squash it forms spaghetti like strands. Besides a marinara sauce or mushroom trio try adding a mixture of cherry tomatoes, Italian parsley, garlic, and touch of lemon juice and extra virgin olive oil to place on top.

**Pumpkin (winter)-**Can be baked and stuffed with your

favorite whole grain rice and bean mixture or diced and added to soups and stews. Save the seeds for roasting as an added treat!

All winter squashes do well on your counter in a cool place for at least a month. Summer squash zucchini and yellow squash need to be refrigerated.

Squashes are great for stuffing with your favorite fillings. Experiment with several combinations of brown rice or other grain and your favorite bean, vegan Italian sausage, onions, and sweet pepper. Squashes are also great diced and added to soups and stews.

## Cruciferous Vegetables

Next on our list of produce to try is cruciferous vegetables. They need their own separate praise for their cancer protective compounds and include the following:

**Cauliflower-** Can be found in a variety of colors such as white, green, purple and orange, can be eaten raw or added to your favorite soups, salad, and stir fry.

**Broccoli-** Broccoli now comes in a variety of colors, white, purple, green, and yellow, can be eaten raw or added to your favorite soups, salad, and stir fry.

**Red Cabbage-** Choose red cabbage over green; both are good for you, but remember the rainbow purple has more antioxidant qualities vs. green. Add cabbage to soups and stews or sauté in your favorite stir fry. Add raw cabbage to salads for a boost to your immune system.

**Bok Choy-** An often-overlooked cruciferous vegetable that is delicious wilted in a stir fry.

**Brussels Sprouts-** Not considered the most loved vegetable by some, but I encourage you try them in different ways. You can steam, roast, and even eat them raw on salads by simply slicing each little cabbage into shreds. Experiment using one of these methods and perhaps you might be astounded that you really do enjoy Brussels sprouts. Avoid boiling vegetables in water as it depletes many of the nutrients. Steaming is quicker and your vegetables will come out delicious and full of flavor. Give Brussels sprouts a second chance as they are a good source of protein, iron, and potassium.

A review of research published in October 1996 issue of the Journal of the American Dietetic Association showed that 70% or more of the studies found a link between cruciferous vegetables and protection against cancer. Cruciferous vegetables fight cancer by reducing oxidative stress, which is an overload of harmful molecules called oxygen free radicals which are generated by our bodies and can be reduced by consuming cruciferous vegetables and reduce the risk of colon, lung, prostate, breast, and other cancers. Ask yourself this: If all it takes is adding vegetables to your diet to help prevent cancer, then why wouldn't you want to add more vegetables to your diet?

## Root Vegetables

Root vegetables are just that: the root of the plant and are high in vitamins and minerals. They absorb their nutrients from the soil. You want to pick ones that are firm not flimsy and free from blemish. If they still have their green tops they should be fresh leaves. Certain root vegetables have unique healing qualities. You may already be familiar with some and others I would encourage you to try for their health benefits.

**Radishes-** They can be found in a variety of colors: red, white, and purple. Radishes are underestimated, maybe because they are so small, but radishes are naturally cooling, making them a great addition to summer meals. They also aid in our digestion by eliminating stagnant food and toxins and they help to prevent viral infections with their high vitamin C and natural cleansing effect on our bodies.

**Beets-** These roots are essential for healthy nerve and muscle function. Beets offer unique health-boosting nutrients you may be missing from your diet.

**Turnips-** This root vegetable is high in water-soluble vitamin C and protects our bodies from the damaging effects of free radicals that can cause inflammation and promotion of cancer.

**Sweet Potatoes-** Here is the perfect prescription for fighting the effects of aging! Sweet potatoes aid in the production of collagen which helps us maintain our skin's youthful elasticity. Better yet, the nutrients in sweet potatoes helps us to cope with stress, while protecting our bodies from cancer, and their high vitamin C helps us to ward off colds and flu viruses. However, you don't want to top them with marshmallows! Better to steam, roast, or bake sweet potatoes.

**Garlic-** This is a plant in the allium (onion) family and throughout ancient history, garlic has been used for its health and medicinal properties. Garlic is known for reducing blood pressure and cholesterol and to combat sickness.

**Rutabaga-** This root is a cross between a turnip and cabbage. It can be added to soups and stews and mashed into potatoes, and its leaves can be used as any green chopped and sautéed for a healthy side dish. It is high in vitamin C and has the ability to boost our immune system, improve our digestive and metabolic health, and build strong bones.

**Celeriac-** Once peeled celeriac is hearty and versatile. It can be boiled, braised, steamed, roasted, or eaten raw in salads. It can be mashed into potatoes or added to soups and stews. It has a nutty, sweet, and delicate celery flavor.

**Carrots-** Beta carotene and fiber are abundant in carrots. Rich in Vitamin A, C, K, B8, pantothenic acid folate, potassium, iron, cooper, and manganese makes it a power food to consume on a daily basis!

**Horseradish-** Adds extra punch to a recipe, but more important with this pungent root vegetable, horseradish has many health benefits associated with it, such as its ability to aid in weight loss, lower blood pressure, help with respiratory ailments, stimulate our digestive system, and improve our immune system.

**Parsnips-** These are closely related to carrots with a slightly sweeter taste. They are high in fiber and vitamins and the high level of potassium makes this root vegetable heart-healthy.

**Daikon Radish-** Is not found in most local grocery stores but can be found in health food markets such as Whole Foods Market and can be found in Asian markets. It is a very large elongated white root. Daikon tastes like a typical red radish only a little sweeter and lighter than standard radishes you are used to consuming. Daikon is known for its great ability to detoxify our bodies. It protects against cancer and boosts our immune system, reduces inflammation, and improves our digestion. You can use daikon raw on salads or added to soups.

**Burdock Root-** This is another one of those unusual root vegetables that you may or may not have had a chance to use. It is used in many types of Asian dishes and can be used peeled or unpeeled. Burdock is known for its liver detoxing ability. It stimulates bile production and digestive juices in the gut, which helps the liver more rapidly process toxins and flush them from our system. Clearing toxins from the blood is one of the main purposes of our liver and consuming burdock root in our cuisine helps us to accomplish this. Burdock root helps with hormonal balance, our skin, and our immune system. There is some caution eating too much burdock root if you are already taking potassium pills. One can get too much of good thing. So, caution is advised to avoid potassium toxicity.

## Consuming the Rainbow

The above list of vegetables will give you plenty of choices to start with when you begin shopping the produce aisle. Bright colors provide a rich diet of the most health-enhancing nutrients our bodies need daily. Shop the rainbow colors, dark rich colors, like orange, red, yellow, and purple.

These intense colors offer even more chemically active antioxidants and pigments than pale ones provide such as:

- Anthocyanidins
- Apigenin
- Hesperetin
- Luteolin
- Par anthocyanidin
- Myricetin
- Quercetin
- Lycopene
- Beta Carotene

Why do antioxidants matter? So-called "free radicals" are small, cell-damaging molecules produced by the body as waste products. Antioxidants neutralize them. Without consuming antioxidants in our diet, we leave our body open to free radicals that attack and damage our cells.

# Fruit, Berries, Nuts & Seeds

Fresh fruit promotes good health; however, you may be asking what about all the fructose? According to studies from the Harvard Health Letter, it isn't naturally-occurring fructose from fruit that is bad for us but the added sugars you are consuming from other products on a daily basis. These added sugars are commonly found in abundance in soft drinks. Sugars are even added to bottled juices and processed foods.

Whole fruit, on the other hand, is beneficial in any amount. Consuming whole fruits has actually shown beneficial to our health by lowering cholesterol, lowering blood pressure, helping with weight loss, and providing our bodies with antioxidants to fight cancer, heart disease, type 2 diabetes, and aging. Most Americans do not consume enough fresh fruit in their daily diets.

Our bodies are an intricate system and thousands of reactions take place in our bodies daily. If you are presently eating a highly-processed and fast food diet you will not be getting the necessary requirements of fiber, nutrients, and antioxidants that our bodies require to work at peak performance. It's not just adults, but children and teens who will purchase an energy bar before choosing a piece of fresh fruit. Energy bars are big business and are misleading in their health benefits as they are usually high in processed sugars. Fresh whole fruit provides instant energy and is a much healthier option.

Americans today are fiber deficient. Fruit adds bulk and fiber to our digestive tract, making elimination easier and more regular. Being constipated in the United Sates is a very big problem and is caused by the lack of fiber in our highly-processed lifestyle and compounded by high meat consumption. You may not realize that fiber only comes from plant foods and is designed by nature to pass through our digestion with ease and helps to keep our bodies healthy. Fiber has few to no calories and promotes a slimmer body by controlling our appetites and keeping our weight in check.

You can buy fresh fruit year-round, making it easy for us to maintain a healthy lifestyle. Some may be seasonal and less expensive if you buy during their peak season.

Most fruits are naturally low in fat, sodium, and calories and contain many essential nutrients that many people are missing from their diets such as potassium, dietary fiber, vitamin C, and folic acid (folate) to name a few. Fruit, melons, citrus, and berries fight cholesterol and helps to prevent heart disease, type 2 diabetes, and cancer. If you are taking medications be aware that some medications can react with certain fruits, check with your doctor or pharmacist if your medication is one of them. Grapefruit is one example that has been known to interact with certain drugs.

## Common Fruits in the USA:

## Winter Fruits

- Cactus Pear
- Clementines
- Date Plums
- Grapefruit
- Kiwifruit
- Mandarin Oranges
- Papaya
- Oranges
- Passion Fruit
- Pear
- Pomegranate
- Tangerines

- Apples

## Spring Fruits

- Apricots
- Barbados Cherries
- Bitter Melon
- Honeydew
- Jackfruit
- Limes
- Lychee (Asian Fruit)
- Mango
- Oranges
- Pineapples
- Strawberries

## Summer Fruits

- Apricots
- Asian Pear
- Barbados Cherries
- Black Currants
- Blackberries
- Blueberries
- Cantaloupe
- Casaba Melon
- Champagne Grapes
- Cherries
- Figs
- Grapes
- Honeydew Melon
- Jackfruit
- Nectarines
- Passion Fruit
- Peaches
- Raspberries
- Strawberries

- Watermelon

## Fall Fruits

- Apples
- Asian Pear
- Cactus Pear
- Cranberries
- Date Plum
- Grapes
- Pear
- Pineapples
- Pomegranate

## Year-Round Fruit

- Apples
- Bananas
- Lemons
- Papayas
- Avocados are actually a fruit. You can find both small and large Hass avocados. Large avocados are great for filling with your favorite whole grain, beans, and veggies. Smaller ones are good for dicing and slicing when called for in a recipe.

## Apples

There are many varieties of apples on the market today and you may want to know which apples are good for baking, snacking, and cooking. It is best to buy your apples organic to avoid unnecessary pesticides. Buying organic will give you peace of mind of not ingesting any more pesticides than necessary; however, if that is not possible, be sure to buy conventional and wash with a vinegar and water solution.

**Braeburn** - Best for snacking; pinkish red apple with a spicy sweet flavor and crisp texture.

**Honey Crisp** - Best or snacking and cooking. Mottled red apples with a sweet mild flavor and a crisp texture.

**Macintosh** - Best for snacking and cooking. Deep red with a green blush. It is tart and tender.

**Cameo** - Best or snacking, baking, and cooking. Red stripes over cream-colored background and has a sweet-tart flavor and crisp texture.

**Jonagold** - Best for snacking, baking, and cooking. Green yellow apple with a red blush and is a sweet tart flavor and a crisp juicy texture.

**Fuji** - Best for snacking. Red and yellow striped apple with a sweet flavor and a crisp texture.

**Gala** - Best for snacking and cooking. It comes in a variety of colors, all with a sweet juicy flavor and crisp and juicy texture.

**Cortland**- Best for snacking, baking, and cooking. Red apple with a sweet tender interior.

**Granny Smith** - Best for snacking, baking, cooking. Green in color; tart, and crisp.

**Rome** - Best for cooking and baking. It is a mildly tart apple.

## Berries are Super Foods!

Just one cup of berries daily can help ward off chronic health conditions. Berries are another great source of incorporating more fiber into our diets. Blueberries, blackberries, raspberries, and strawberries are rich in nutrients, antioxidants, and phytochemicals, which may help to prevent and in some cases even reverse the effects of aging, heart disease, arthritis, diabetes, and certain cancers. Raspberries contain ellagic acid a compound with anti-cancer properties. Blueberries are believed to contain the highest antioxidant capacity of all commonly consumed fruits and vegetables. They contain polyphenols called flavonoids, and one in particular is anthocyanins, which is a type of antioxidant found in berries that give berries their dark color and fight the effects of free radicals on cells.

Many people avoid buying berries because of their short freshness cycle when brought home from the market. A good tip for storing all your berries is to store them in a mason jar or any glass jar with a lid. Do not wash them. Place the jars in your refrigerator and only wash them when you are ready to consume them. They will stay fresh for a week or longer.

Berries are a perfect addition to add to your salads or on your favorite whole grain cereal or dairy free yogurt. Add berries to your favorite smoothie or try freezing different berries into ice cubes to add to your water and ice teas for a fruit flavor.

When purchasing berries at your market try to choose berries that are plump, tender, and bright in color. Avoid containers that are damp or stained, which might be an indication of overripe fruit.

## Citrus Benefits

Citrus fruits include oranges, lemons, limes, and grapefruits in addition to tangerines and pomelos. These are our go-to fruits for Vitamin C, which is a powerful antioxidant protecting our bodies from the dangers of free radicals. Vitamin C is required by our bodies for the synthesis of collagen which helps wounds to heal. Collagen helps hold our blood vessels, tendons, ligaments, and bone together. Studies have shown that citrus may improve blood flow through coronary arteries and may reduce blood clots and prevent LDL or bad cholesterol which causes arterial plaques. If you are taking medications check with your pharmacist or doctor to be sure there is no interaction with consuming citrus and your medications.

Try a squeeze of lemon or lime for adding a zesty flavor to all your favorite dishes and salads or add lemon or lime juice to your water for a refreshing drink. Make a fruit Buddha bowl with orange and grapefruit slices, a ½ cup of brown rice and ½ cup of non-dairy plain yogurt and top with a drizzle of honey and sprinkle of nuts or seeds. Your body will thank you for it!

## The Benefits of Melons

**Cantaloupe** is high in essential vitamins and minerals and make for an easy snack that is low in fat and has no cholesterol, while supplying our bodies with Vitamin C, which helps to maintain all of our body tissues. Cantaloupe is high in Vitamin A. A deficiency of vitamin A may lead to a poorly functioning immune system. Our eyes are important and Vitamin A will help us achieve good retinal health.

**Honeydew Melon** like the watermelon honeydew melon has a high-water content and potassium, making it a great choice for maintaining healthy blood pressure levels. Honeydews also contain Vitamin C and copper and aiding collagen production and tissue repair and are also a good source of B vitamins which helps to remove toxins that can cause illness and disease.

**Watermelon**: what better way to refresh us on a hot summer day than to eat watermelon! Watermelon is mostly water, in fact, 92% water! Watermelon contains beta carotene and lycopene, combating the effects of free radicals in our cells. Health benefits include prevention of kidney disorders, high blood pressure and aids in the prevention of cancer, heart disease, diabetes, heat stroke, macular degeneration, and impotence. Eating a little bit of that rind supplies fiber as well.

Although they may seem seasonal I have found tasty melons year-round. If you happen to buy one and it seems flavorless, most grocery stores will let you return it for a refund or to exchange it for another one.

# Nuts and Seeds

Are nuts and seeds good for us? Yes, yes, yes, but in moderation. Nuts and seeds are typically high in natural oil and calories. One handful a day will be plenty to help us maintain our health and satisfy those tricky cravings you may have in between meals.

A handful of nuts can help improve our cholesterol, keep blood sugar levels stable, and help in reducing heart disease. Nuts have fiber, magnesium, and potassium and B6 for heart disease protection. Certain nuts and seeds contain Omega 3 such as walnuts, chia seeds, flax seeds and hemp seeds which help reduce inflammation in our bodies. All nuts and seeds are rich in vitamin E, an antioxidant that helps maintain healthy skin and eyes. Brazil nuts are high in selenium and zinc, B6 and biotin, which benefits not only healthy skin but also in keeping our nails and hair healthy. Best of all, nuts and seeds add protein into our diets and are a cancer-fighting food. Compounds like carotene, resveratrol, lutein, and cryptoxanthin found in nuts and seeds help protect us against cancer, heart disease, degenerative nerve disease, Alzheimer's disease, diabetes, and viral/fungal infections.

Unfortunately, many people avoid eating nuts and seeds as they are afraid they will gain weight, but that might only happen if you overindulge in eating nuts. Nuts and seeds are your companions. You can carry them along with you at school, work, or play. They are a great road trip snack and are easy to store in small containers. They have a long shelf life if stored properly in your refrigerator or freezer, which prevents them from going rancid.

Nuts and seeds have long been admired in many culinary dishes. They can also be roasted and spiced for added flavor to dishes and enjoyed in baked breads and muffins or just eaten by the handful.

You can find them salted for snacking and unsalted for using in your favorite dessert or main dish. You can find many recipes online using cashews to make a wonderful non-dairy cream cheese, sour cream, and yogurt. Try making your own healthy granola cereal using oats, nuts, seeds, and dried fruits.

Here is a list of nuts and seeds you might want to add to your grocery list:

***Nuts-***
- Almonds
- Walnuts
- Brazil Nuts
- Cashews
- Pecans
- Macadamia Nuts
- Pistachio
- Pine nuts

***Seeds-***
- Sunflower
- Pumpkin
- Chia
- Flax
- Sesame
- Hemp

Tip: Store nuts and seeds in the refrigerator or freezer to keep them fresh longer.

## Sprouting

Many of us have already seen sprouts in our grocery store. You might see mung bean sprouts for making stir-fries and Asian dishes and you may see alfalfa or broccoli sprouts to add to sandwiches and salads. A new hobby is sprouting your own seeds. There are several techniques online for sprouting your own seeds at home. Mason jars with lids specific for sprouting can be found online and in some health food stores and for the serious sprouter there are electric sprouters that automatically water your sprouts which leaves the task of daily washing and adding new water to a mason jar no longer necessary. However, if you are new to sprouting the mason jar technique is far less expensive and best for beginners.

If you are curious enough to grow your own sprouts, there are many online sites and health food stores that sell organic seeds for you to experiment with. There are many inexpensive varieties and mixes from which to choose. Sprouts provide a significant number of vitamins, enzymes, and nutrients to your body. They have the ability to improve digestion, boost our metabolism, and increase enzymatic activity throughout our bodies while supporting our immune systems.

Sprouting is like having a mini garden in your kitchen. The process of changing little seeds into little plants is easy, but the benefits of consuming these sprouts are tremendous!

So, what happens when you sprout beans, seeds, and grains? When you soak, and sprout your beans, seeds or grains it lowers the amount of phytic acid, which can bind to minerals and lead to mineral deficiency. Phytic acid is found within the hulls of many grains as well as legumes of various types. Sprouting reduces the amount of phytic acid, however, some still remains.

Some believe that sprouts contain a *life force* due to their high enzymes and protein content. For some who may have a problem digesting certain grains, beans, and legumes, sprouting may help to make them more digestible. Alfalfa seeds, broccoli seeds, and mung beans are easy to grow and are a great addition to your salads.

If you like to be adventurous in your kitchen give sprouting a try and see if you like it, otherwise, just buy and enjoy them from the store!

# Spices and Herbs

You may not think about all the health benefits you may already have in your pantry in the form of spices. A spice is a seed, fruit, root, bark, berry, bud, or vegetable and is added to food for flavoring or coloring.

Spices have long been known for their health benefits. They help to reduce LDL bad cholesterol and are known for their antioxidants. They are antimicrobial and help to shield our body from free radical damage, while being anti-inflammatory.

Some of the most common spices used in many plant-based recipes are cloves, cinnamon, allspice, saffron, fennel, oregano, cumin, garlic, mustard, turmeric, ginger, red pepper and black pepper, paprika, curry powders, garam masala, coriander seeds, and cardamom. Experiment with different spices in all your recipes and baked goods. Keep in mind a little goes a long way as spices tend to have a robust flavor and could overpower your recipe.

Turmeric teas are now touted as the new health drink. Turmeric tea recipes can be consumed hot or cold. It is delicious, with a unique flavor, and has the added anti-inflammatory benefit to reduce inflammation, reduce joint and muscle pain, lower blood sugar, renew our skin and may even help with depression. Simply add water to an 8-ounce glass if drinking cold or fill your tea cup with hot water. Add 1 tsp. of turmeric paste (turmeric and dab of water mixed into a paste) to your glass or cup. Add a squeeze of lemon juice and 1-2 T. of organic raw honey. Mix and enjoy!

Culinary Herbs are anti-inflammatory, anti-bacterial, anti-fungal, anti-parasitic while offering us vitamins and minerals. Herbs can be antiseptic, diuretic, blood purifiers, and some can detox our bodies of heavy metals.

Fresh herbs are wonderful, but it is also good to have dried herbs on hand when fresh are not available. Look for basil, chives, cilantro, garlic, ginger, mint, oregano, parsley, rosemary and thyme. Growing your own fresh herbs is fun and if you own a dehydrator as I do, you can dehydrate your fresh herbs, and grind them in a coffee grinder or blender, then store in sealed mason jars.

I have also bought fresh bay leaves from Asian Markets and dehydrate them. They are so much fresher and greener to use in soups and stews. Grow fresh herbs in your kitchen, which not only smell wonderful but are handy when called for in a recipe. One doesn't need a large area to grow fresh herbs, any window sill or patio porch will work. If you were like me growing up, I used spices and herbs because a recipe may have called for it, not even thinking about all the health benefits they were providing.

We need to look at food differently from now on by training our minds to recognize the difference of eating processed foods vs. fresh whole foods and what it may be doing to our bodies. Every time you consume a food product you will learn to ask yourself, how is this going to benefit my body? If the food item in question doesn't have a benefit, you will learn to set it aside.

# Plant-Based Protein

Today Americans are consuming a high amount of animal protein in their diets. Research studies have concluded this level of animal protein is having adverse effects in our health and causing a host of illnesses that can be corrected if not even reversed by just switching animal protein to plant protein, which, by the way, is better utilized by our bodies. It surprises many to learn that even vegetables have protein such as broccoli and potatoes and don't forget Popeye and eat your spinach! One cannot be protein deficient on a plant-based diet.

Besides vegetables, beans, and legumes there are three other plant-based meat alternatives that are used quite often when transitioning from an animal based diet to a plant-based diet. Tofu, tempeh (a fermented soy and probiotic good for digestive health) and seitan also known as "wheat meat". Contrary to many TV shows making fun of tofu and perhaps giving it a bad name, knowing how to properly prepare tofu can provide a nutritious and delicious meal.

There are also many transitional meat analogues on the market such as chicken, beef, pork, and fish that taste good and their texture mimics real meat, but because they are plant proteins these meat analogues are void of the fat and cholesterol found in animal based foods and offer fiber and other nutrients lacking in an animal based diet.

When you change to a plant-based diet and stop eating the animal protein in meat, fish, dairy, and eggs, you will soon notice your taste buds change and foods take on a more vibrant and delicious flavor.

There are many temptations in our grocery stores that might make the right food choices difficult. It is a challenge, but it's a choice between wanting to be healthy or sick; living or dying. Most people today are sick of being sick whether it's a major illness or just plain everyday ills, like headaches, fatigue, allergies, colds, and flu. Being sick tells us our immune system is out of balance. The way to optimize our health and to fight these illnesses is to feed our bodies with whole foods that will nourish us and promote good health.

Some may worry that B12 is missing from their diet because they no longer are consuming meat; however, you can find many vegan products enriched with B12 and other vitamins. Many on a vegan diet take a supplemental B12 to allay any fears of deficiency.

B12 is synthesized by soil bacteria. We consume B-12 by eating the meat from the cow which has grazed in pastures. As animals eat plant material, some of the attached dirt is ingested along with the bacterial growth, however, we need to realize that meat products available today in most grocery stores are not derived from grazing animals. Most meat is from animals that are raised on grains and treated with chemicals/drugs that destroy most bacterial growth. That being said, many people may be deficient in B-12 whether you eat meat or not.

## Beans and Legumes

Protein is found in plants. Beans and legumes are one of four great sources of plant protein without the saturated fat and cholesterol that comes from eating animal protein. Beans and Legumes are great choice for protein in our diets with an added bonus of minerals and fiber. Many people avoid beans due to the unfavorable side effect of gas, but the more you eat them the better your body begins to digest them, and it soon will balance out. Remember: most Americans are fiber-deficient and just adding healthy foods to their diets will help them with elimination and cleaning out their bowels, which may have been backed up for years.

Did you know that just three ounces of black beans has 24 grams of protein and is only 120 calories with the added benefit of lower acidity, no cholesterol, no saturated fat, 9 grams of fiber and phytonutrients? Four ounces of ground beef has 24-gram protein and 320 calories with few health benefits. Eating meat increases acidity, cholesterol, and saturated fat, with no fiber. Meat also contains heterocyclic amines. These HCAs are compounds that are released when meat is cooked at high temperatures (exceeding 300 degrees) such as grilling, broiling and even pan frying and creating carcinogenic substances. The math is easy on which is better for you: black beans or meat.

Let's take a look at the benefits of adding more beans to your diet. Beans contain soluble fiber and saponins and phytosterols, which help lower our bad, LDL, cholesterol. Just ½ – 1 ½ cup of beans daily may help reduce blood cholesterol levels.

Many people are constantly hungry. Eating beans will help you feel fuller longer and they have a slower rise in blood sugar levels while giving you a steady flow of energy throughout your day. They are a complex carbohydrate supper food providing a steady source of good glucose instead of eating a simple carbohydrate that causes the up and down spikes of blood sugar and feelings of fatigue throughout your day.

Reducing flatulence is something people are concerned about when consuming beans. You may reduce this issue by being sure to rinse your beans if they're coming from a can or changing the soaking water several times when using dried beans. Adding a bay leaf or sprinkle of caraway seeds may help to ease flatulence. You can also buy a product called Beano that may help until your body adjusts to eating beans.

When cooking dried beans, add salt *after* your beans have cooked, not before, as the salt will prevent beans from cooking properly. Some people may find cooking dried beans inconvenient; however, using a pressure cooker works wonders, especially if you forget to soak your beans overnight. I always like to keep a few canned beans on hand for those days you just don't feel like cooking. Of course, canned beans are always great to keep on hand during weather emergencies and loss of electrical power.

Beans are not only tasty and high in protein but they are an inexpensive food you can add to all your favorite dishes. Beans go well in soups and stews and are great on salads or used in a tortilla for a fantastic wrap.

Add these beans to your grocery list:

- Black Beans- Great added to Mexican cuisine
- Red Bean - Great on salads and added to soups and stews
- Kidney Beans-Great on salads and added to soups and stews
- Cannellini Beans- Great for Italian cuisine
- Navy Beans- Great for Italian cuisine
- Garbanzo Beans- Great for Mediterranean dishes and Indian cuisine
- Pinto Beans- Great for Mexican and tropical cuisine
- Edamame Beans- Great added to a stir-fry and Asian cuisine
- Fresh Green Beans- Good in soups and stews and bean salads or vegetable stir-fry
- Fresh Yellow Beans- Good in soups and stews and bean salads or vegetable stir-fry
- Hummus- is made from chickpeas and is great as a spread on veggie wraps in place of vegan mayo.

Lentils are legumes. They are very tiny seeds that grow in pods and may be either round or oval in shape. They come in different colors of brown, red, or green. Green Lentils hold up best in cooking. Lentils are known, like beans, to lower cholesterol and help manage blood sugar levels. Lentils are high in fiber and are an excellent source of minerals, vitamins, and protein with virtually no fat. Lentils are a good source of folic acid and magnesium. Studies show that a deficiency of magnesium is associated with a heart attack and free radical injury to our hearts following a heart attack. Lentils are a complex carbohydrate, increasing energy and help to replace our iron stores.

Lentils can be found canned or in dry packages at your grocery store. I would recommend with all canned items that you look for cans marked BPA-FREE, as there is a potential health concern for food in cans that contain bisphenol A/BPA linings. Eden is one brand whose cans are BPA-free, but more and more companies are packaging BPA-free cans or packaging their "canned" foods in boxes to avoid this health hazard.

Lentils are quick and easy and cook in around 20 minutes (firmer consistency) and unlike dried beans they do not need to be soaked ahead of time. If making Indian cuisine where your dish requires a softer consistency you can cook them an additional 10-15 minutes. Lentils make for a wonderful replacement in meat dishes like shepherd's pie and are delicious in salads seasoned with your favorite herbs and added to any of your favorite soup and stew recipes.

Lentils like beans contain purines, which for some individuals can cause health problems. Please check with your doctor if you have concerns whether lentils can be added to your diet.

Scientific research suggests that consuming beans and lentils may help prevent certain types of cancer such as estrogen type cancers, pancreatic cancer, colon cancer, breast cancer, and prostate cancers. Beans contain both lignin and phytates which appear to be beneficial for fighting cancer. Beans help you to feel full and they add fiber to your diet without all of the calories, helping with weight reduction. Beans contain soluble fiber and help to stabilize blood sugar spikes while providing us with a lasting source of energy from complex carbohydrates and proteins to keep our bodies working at peak performance levels. Beans are also heart-healthy by reducing our cholesterol as they do not contain saturated fat and consuming beans will help to raise our good HDL while keeping your bad LDL levels down.

## Tempeh

Tempeh is made from fermented soybeans. It has a distinct flavor. Steaming tempeh helps to lighten the fermented flavor and leaves you with a pleasant nutty flavor. Steam tempeh for approximately 10-15 minutes before adding any marinades or before using it in dishes.

Crumble tempeh and use it in recipes as a hamburger replacement. Use tempeh to replace chicken in a wonderful no-chicken salad sandwich. Tempeh can be sliced or diced and used in a stir fry and is a great bacon replacement. You can find tempeh bacon in your grocery stores.

## Tofu

Tofu is a curd made from soybeans. Tofu has a mild taste and alone has little flavor. This feature makes creating recipes with tofu wonderful as it will pick up on the flavor of whatever dish you are creating. Like meat, tofu may also be marinated with seasonings, spices, and flavorings, to enhance its flavor. Tofu is now found in most grocery stores and almost all health food stores. There are two types: refrigerated vacuumed sealed and shelf-stable. Both are basically the same but may vary in texture and preferred use.

There are several choices and to be successful using tofu you need to understand all the varieties out there. First and foremost is knowing the different textures. There is extra firm, firm, and soft. Vacuumed sealed is found in the refrigerated section of your grocery store. It must be kept cold and remain in the liquid until ready to use. Vacuumed sealed is best for baking, broiling, and pan frying. Extra firm and firm works best for these cooking methods.

Silken tofu, on the other hand, is shelf stable and comes in a small box and no refrigeration is necessary until it is opened. Silken tofu can also be purchased soft, firm, or extra firm. Soft and silken tofu are best used for sauces and desserts and sometimes used in soups such as miso soup.

Many recipes call for draining vacuumed sealed tofu twice. Once from the liquid it contains inside the box and a second pressing using the following technique:

1. Layer 2-3 paper towels on a dish or pan that has an edge.
2. Next, place your block of tofu on the paper towel. You can also slice the block of tofu into 3 slices rather than leave in one large block for quicker draining.
3. Place several paper towels on top of your tofu block or slices and place a lint free towel on top of paper towels.
4. Place a second plate or pan on top of your final wrapped tofu block or slices and place a heavy

object on the dish or pan, which will weigh down on the tofu and help release as much liquid from the tofu as possible.

This pressing is necessary as it can release as much as ½ cup more liquid from the tofu. Omitting this process will make it difficult to bake, grill, or sauté your tofu.

There are several gadgets online at Amazon.com under tofu presses; some more expensive than others and can make pressing tofu a lot easier and quicker. Tofu Express is one such device that does all the work for you quickly.

If pan frying your tofu, dust it with seasoned non-GMO cornstarch on both sides. This will create a light golden crust on the outside while keeping the tofu soft on the inside. Most recipes will tell you which tofu to use for best results, such as vacuumed sealed or silken and extra-firm, firm, or soft.

Butler Soy Curls- This is an interesting meat alternative that is fun to work with. It is a soy product you can order online at Butler Soy Curls. This product requires rehydration and is used in many dishes to replace chicken, beef, or pork. They are delicious when combined with your favorite sauces. Soy curls are non-GMO and a great option for those who are gluten intolerant and cannot consume seitan, which is a wheat product. Try their vegan jerky; it is spicy and very tasty and great to carry in your backpack if hiking or taking a road trip.

## Seitan

Seitan, also known as wheat gluten, wheat meat, or wheat protein, is a favorite meat substitute in a plant-based diet as it mimics meat in texture and taste when mixed with your favorite sauce, spice, or herb. This is a wheat product. Anyone who is suffering from celiac disease or may be gluten sensitive would want to avoid seitan in your diet. For those who can eat gluten, seitan makes a wonderful meat alternative and can be made into a roast, rolled into sausages, and shaped into cutlets.

You might want to experiment with the many prepared meat alternatives on the market today that are made with wheat gluten and other plant based proteins. Tofurky, Field Roast, Gardein, and Lightlife offer a variety of choices such as beefless chunks for stews and pot roast, chicken and turk'y varieties. You can even find fishless fillets and crabless cakes available from Gardein. Tofurky and Lightlife offer sausages, frankfurters, and lunchmeat. Beyond Meat and a few Gardein products offer gluten-free options.

Nutritionally, seitan is a powerhouse of good solid protein equivalent to a steak, but with no saturated fat or cholesterol, making it a perfect meat alternative. Seitan can be purchased readymade and sold as chunks or strips by West Soy. You may find it already marinated and ready to heat or original flavor or chick'n flavor so you can add your own favorite sauce or flavoring.

At first you may find consuming meat alternatives a bit different then real meat. You must realize they are meant to mimic meat in taste and texture. Meat analogues will also help those who find it hard to give up meat an easier transition to enjoying a plant-based diet.

It takes about 30 days for our taste buds to change; most are replaced in about 15 days. You will find as you eat more plant based foods, things will taste cleaner and more vibrant as you eliminate more of the animal fats from your diet.

# Mushrooms

Mushrooms are a fungus and a great vegan meat alternative. Not only are they delicious, but they offer many health benefits. Crimini, oyster, portobello, shiitake, or white button are common mushrooms found in most grocery stores. Mushrooms are loaded with essential nutrients. Mushrooms contain selenium, which is a mineral found in the soil and plays a key role in our metabolism, boosts our immune function, and provides our bodies with antioxidants that help fight those nasty free radicals that can damage our cells. Mushrooms contain B vitamins which turns carbohydrates into fuel and helps our body to metabolize fats and protein.

When exposed to sunlight (ultraviolet B, or UVB light), mushrooms convert ergosterol (a naturally occurring compound in mushrooms) into an active form of Vitamin D. Sources from the Mayo Clinic state that fungus is the only food source of vitamin D besides animal products. No other plants provide vitamin D and the B-12 found naturally in mushrooms is the same as found in meat.

The meaty savory flavor of mushrooms can be as satisfying in a recipe as meat, offering far fewer calories from fat that one gets from consuming meat. An example would be pot roast made with mushrooms in place of beef or mushroom stroganoff. Large portobello mushrooms can be a hamburger replacement topped with all your favorite toppings, such as lettuce, onions, and tomatoes. Don't forget: large portobello are great stuffed with whole grains and veggies and who would have thought that sliced and sautéed mushrooms can replace bacon in your diet, avoiding all the fat and nitrates known to be dangerous to our health that come with eating real bacon. Mushrooms are a win-win!

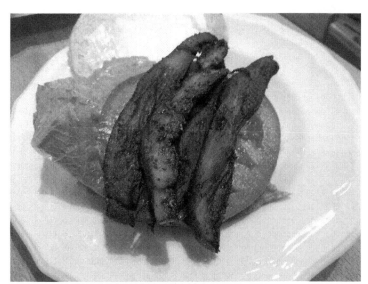

**Portobello Mushroom Bacon**

# Fermented Foods

## Gut Health

When your gut health is not working properly it can cause a host of problems such as bloating, gas, diarrhea, and stomach pain. Our gut health plays a huge role in why we feel sick. It may show up as hormonal imbalances, autoimmune illness, diabetes, fibromyalgia, chronic fatigue, and skin rashes. In order to recover our gut to a healthy state consider a plant-based diet, which reduces inflammatory foods from our diet. Some may need to do a temporary elimination diet from foods they may be sensitive to such as gluten or wheat. Infections from parasites, yeast, and bacteria can also play havoc on gut health.

A plant-based diet can help with many symptoms associated with an unhealthy gut and may avoid an appointment with a gastroenterologist to repair any health issues you may be experiencing.

## Prebiotics

Prebiotics are just as important as probiotics for gut health and are the fuel for our good bacteria to grow. This healthy microbiome is our defense system against toxins we encounter daily from the consumption of animal products, environment, consuming poor quality tap water, and common yeast and viruses.

Prebiotics are easily found and consumed on a plant-based diet taking any guess work away if we are getting the necessary prebiotics in our diet. A plant-based diet provides our bodies with a steady flow of nutrient-dense prebiotic foods.

- Beans
- Bananas

- Asparagus
- Onions
- Garlic
- Cabbage

## Probiotics

Probiotics are good bacteria. They provide live bacteria and yeast that promote a healthy digestive system. Probiotics help common conditions, such as irritable bowel syndrome, inflammatory bowel disease, and infectious diarrhea that may be caused by a virus, bacteria, or parasite. When may our probiotics be in danger? Overuse of antibiotics is one example and one that is often abused by many who feel an antibiotic will cure everything. A plant-based diet offers both prebiotic and probiotic health and will certainly reduce, eliminate, and outperform your need for antibiotics.

Probiotics are fermented foods and can be consumed in several different ways. As many probiotics contain dairy, we will be looking at non-dairy probiotics allowed on a plant-based diet.

*Sauerkraut-* Unpasteurized or homemade is best. Great as a side dish or served on a veggie hot dog or hamburger.

Kimchi- Is a spicy Korean fermented cabbage. Some kimchi found in stores may have seafood in the ingredients, which is not allowed on a plant-based diet. Be sure to check ingredient labels.

*Tempeh-* Is a fermented tofu derived from soybeans. It is a much firmer texture than tofu and is great used as ground crumbles to replace any ground beef dishes. You can find tempeh in most grocery stores now; some are already marinated or bacon flavored.

*Sourdough Bread-* A probiotic-friendly and great-tasting bread that is dairy- and egg-free.

*Sour Pickles-*Dill and sour pickles are both great sources of probiotics.

*Olives-* Usually come in a briny water and are an easy way to add probiotics to our diet.

*Kombucha-* Is a fermented drink and can be easily found in most supermarkets or you can make your own. Kombucha has active enzymes, antioxidants, amino acids and probiotics. It is a mixture of black or green tea and cane sugar and is then fermented by bacteria and yeast commonly known as a SCOBY (symbiotic colony of bacteria and yeast). Drinking kombucha tea provides our bodies with probiotics along with many other tremendous health benefits. You can now find this drink in many grocery stores. If you want to learn about making your own kombucha tea there are many internet sites with directions.

*Miso-* Is a fermented soy paste. Typically, miso is made from a mixture of soybeans, sea salt and rice koji (aspergillus culture added to steamed soya beans) that is then fermented. The fermentation creates enzyme-rich compounds that are effective in detoxifying the body, eliminating industrial pollution, radioactivity, and artificial chemicals found in many foods.

Miso is a wonderful sweet or savory paste that is salty in flavor. It comes in a deep red or dark color with earthy tones and hearty flavor for adding to hearty stews and soups during the fall and winter months and light and sweet tasting for soups and stews in the spring and summer months. If adding to your soup or stew always add miso as the last ingredient as accidental boiling of miso will kill all the healthy benefits. Best to add miso once your soup or stew pot is off your heat source or you can add your miso paste to individual soup bowls (1/2 tsp. per bowl) followed by your soup or stew.

Miso soup has long been recognized by the macrobiotic diet and studies have shown that this fermented soy paste may reduce one's risk of cancer; including breast, prostate, lung, and colon cancers. It is antiviral and very alkalizing and strengthening to our immune system. Miso contains all essential amino acids which makes it a complete protein and a good plant based source to restore beneficial probiotics to the intestines.

# The War on Dairy

We're all familiar with TV ads touting the milk mustache and that cheese and real butter are good for us, but are they really? Millions of adults and children are lactose intolerant and cannot digest the proteins found in milk. These advertisements on TV and in magazines have led us to believe that dairy is required for healthy bones and we need the calcium from dairy to protect us from hip fractures and to improve our bone density. How many of you have researched and found just the opposite is happening to our bodies when dairy is consumed? To be honest with you there is more scientific research against consuming dairy than to consume dairy products as recommended by the FDA.

In research studies across the country, dairy has been linked to an increase cancer. Casein, a natural protein found in dairy, has been shown in laboratory studies to increase the risk of cancer cell tumor growth raising IGF-1 factors (insulin-like growth factors) and linked to estrogen type cancers such as colon, breast, ovarian, and prostate cancers. Other research studies have shown a possibility that dairy may contribute to type 1 diabetes through a process called molecular mimicry. Multiple sclerosis has been linked to high dairy consumption and increased high cholesterol and atherosclerosis in studies. What is concerning is that 71% of Americans use milk as their go-to protein. Be aware there are two types of protein found in dairy: *casein* and *whey* protein. Thirty eight percent of the solid matter in milk consists of 80% casein and 20% whey. Casein is the main ingredient in all cheese after the liquid has been strained away. Whey and casein are digested differently in the body. Whey is more quickly absorbed by way of the bloodstream, raising insulin and casein stimulating our insulin growth factor IGF-1 which in studies increases our risk of cancer cell tumor growth.

It appears that dairy and cheese are probably the most difficult to give up on a plant-based diet. One may ask why this is? Dr. T. Colin Campbell, professor emeritus at Cornell university and author of *The China Study*, found casein to be the most relevant cancer promoter ever discovered! Casein digests very slowly and contains a substance called casomorphin which is a natural morphine-like substance and acts like opiates in our body. Casein breaks down in the stomach, producing the peptide casomorphin, which is an opioid but also acts as a histamine releaser, which is also why so many people are allergic to dairy products. Casomorphins create such an addictive response that it has been compared to the strength of heroine, causing food additions and mood disorders. No wonder we all loved cheese!

Other symptoms people experience with dairy may be excess mucus, respiratory problems, digestive issues such as constipation and diarrhea, rashes, acne and skin irritations. Dairy is not a health food by any means and should be avoided and all cost.

There are many non-dairy products that are very good to replace the dairy in your life. Non-dairy milk is inexpensive and there are several varieties, such as non-GMO soy milk, almond milk, cashew milk, oat milk, rice milk, coconut milk, flax-seed milk, and many more. Non-dairy ice cream, sour cream, and cream cheese can also be found. Each state usually carries their own brand of non-dairy food items. Ask customer service if you have trouble finding non-dairy products at your market. Health food stores and groceries stores like Whole Foods Market carry *Soyatoo Soy* or *Rice* whipping cream and *So Delicious* makes a coconut whipped cream. Butter choices are *Earth Balance* or organic non-GMO *Smart Balance*. Non-dairy yogurt is available both plain unsweetened or fruit flavored and sweetened. *Daiya* products include sliced cheese, blocked cheese, and shredded cheese. They also offer flavored cream cheeses. *Follow Your Heart* has a huge selection of vegan cheese, mayonnaise, creamy salad dressing, tartar sauce, and horseradish mayo that are all delicious! There are also many recipes online and in vegan cookbooks for making tofu ricotta cheese. *So Delicious* makes a wonderful ice creams that are coconut-based, almond-based, or soy-based. *Ben and Jerry's* also makes a marvelous non-dairy ice cream (Note: it is usually located next to their whole milk ice cream so be sure to check the front label for the words "non-dairy").

There are many recipes and cookbooks that even show us how to make our own non-dairy recipes using cashews to make delicious cheese or butter, ice cream, mayonnaise, milk, and creamers. Most are easy to make, but some do require kitchen equipment to make them such as a Vita Mix, Blend Tec, blender, stand mixer, or food processor.

# To Oil or Not to Oil

There is some controversy on whether oil is good or bad for us. If you have read the studies and research of plant-based authors such as T. Colin Campbell, Dr. Neal Barnard, Dr. Caldwell Esselstyn, Dr. Dean Ornish, Dr. Joel Fuhrman, and Dr. John A. McDougall you know they all recommend no oils. Oils, whether they be monounsaturated and polyunsaturated, coconut, or cold pressed, are considered a processed food with no nutritional value and empty calories. Studies have shown that even the highest quality of oils should be avoided since they may cause damage to our arteries, increase our blood pressure, hinder weight loss goals, and increase ill health.

Our brain's overall composition is 50-60% pure fat and the rest a combination of protein and carbohydrates. Our brain needs fat as it insulates our brain nerve cells. How much fat do we need then and in what form? Males need 12-16% and Females 18-24%. We want to strive to consume good fats in their *natural* state such as walnuts, avocados, nuts, seeds, and olives in moderation, as these healthy fats not only help our joints and nerves, but contain antioxidants that help to lower our risk for heart disease, high cholesterol, and lower blood pressure. We don't by any means want to be fat-free. We do need fats in our diets as they are important in the digestion of fat soluble vitamins A, K, D, and E and are vital to our health.

Research has shown that *all* processed oils may contribute to an increase in HDL bad cholesterol keeping our health at risk for heart disease as well as keeping us from our desired weight loss goals. There are many books by renowned doctors; as mentioned above, they have written several books regarding the use of oil in our diets. You may want to investigate their findings in more detail by visiting their websites or reading their books.

An easy and healthier substitute for oil is obtaining our fat from whole natural plant sources such as avocados, nuts, and seeds and olives. Substitute water or vegetable broth in place of oil when cooking.

## Omega 3 Fatty Acids

Omega 3 fatty acid is often a concern on a plant based diet. Omega 3s are essential fats that our bodies can't make on their own and must be obtained from the foods we consume. Omega 3 fats are derived from alpha-linolenic acid ALA which is converted into EPA and DHA. Omega-3s are used in the formation of cell walls and assist in improving our circulation and oxygen intake. Research shows that omega 3 fatty acids reduce inflammation and may lower our risk for chronic diseases such as heart disease, cancer, and arthritis.

Unfortunately, the Standard American Diet and over-consumption of processed foods contain more Omega-6 fatty acids in our diet and is creating inflammation in our bodies. We are told by our doctors and in advertising that to improve our intake of Omega-3 people should be consuming fish or taking fish supplements; however, today our fish may not contain the omega-3 as we once thought due to the extreme pollution in our waters. Mercury from fish is also a concern and in high consumption can be toxic and harmful to our health. It is better to obtain our omega-3 in plant form such as flax meal, hempseeds, nuts (walnuts are best), leafy vegetables, edamame (fresh soybeans), black beans, kidney beans, and winter squashes. If you still feel you may need an additional boost there are many vegan omega-3 supplements made from plant sources you can order online.

# Mastering the Art of Baking

Mastering the art of vegan baking is quite easy. In fact, most cookie and cake recipes seldom need a mixer. Vegan baking requires a few substitutions, for example, eggs, dairy, cream cheese, or yogurt are easily replaced with the same ingredients called for, but using non-dairy substitutions. Even though vegan baking is healthier in the long run as we are eliminating the cholesterol, high fructose corn syrup, and hydrogenated oils, they still have empty calories that offer no health benefit. It is best to limit these empty calories and save desserts for special occasions and holidays. Too many of us have a birthday celebration every day! Store bought desserts may contain genetically modified ingredients (unless labeled non-GMO) and more than likely will contain high fructose corn syrup and hydrogenated oils, which we are trying to avoid.

## Non-Dairy Baking Ingredients:

- Non-Dairy Soy, Almond or Coconut Milk
- Earth Balance or organic Non-GMO Smart Balance
- Vegan Sour Cream- Follow Your Heart Brand
- Vegan Cream Cheese- Follow Your Heart Brand
- Non-Dairy Yogurt- baking usually uses plain and unsweetened
- Non-Dairy Whipped Cream
- Silken tofu

Soy, almond, and coconut milk are best for baking. Soy milk is similar to whole milk, almond milk will impart a little nutty flavor, and coconut milk would give a slight coconut flavor. I have had success using both unsweetened and sweetened, as well as plain or vanilla flavored non-dairy milks in baking with no issues.

## Replacing Eggs

Eggs are easily replaced by the following choices:

- 1 ½ tsp. of Ener-G Foods Egg Replacer + 2 T. lukewarm water = 1 egg (whisk into a froth)
- 1 T. Ground Flaxseed meal + 3 T. water = 1 egg (Mix together and set aside until it gels in about 5 minutes)
- 2 Tsp. of whole psyllium husk + 3 T. water + 1 ½ tsp. of neutral vegetable oil = 1 egg (mix together and set aside for a few minutes to gel). Whole psyllium husk can be ordered online through Amazon.
- 2 Level T. of VeganEgg (by Follow Your Heart) + 1/2 cup of cold water = 1 Egg (whisk powder and water together)

Many baking recipes call for a neutral oil such as non-GMO cold-pressed canola oil, refined coconut oil (no coconut flavor) or unrefined (if you want a coconut flavor) or grapeseed oil. *Remember: if you prefer not to use oils, you can replace them with the same ratio using organic applesauce.* Applesauce found in multi-packs are perfect as most recipes call for 1/3 cup of oil and one container of applesauce is about 1/3 cup.

Icing and frostings call for shortening or vegan butter. Spectrum organic shortening contains no hydrogenated oils. You can use either Earth Balance or Smart Balance butter.

## Sugar

Everyone loves sweets and unfortunately sugar is sugar. Look for natural organic sugars. Florida Crystals, found in most markets are vegan. If you are following a vegan recipe for baking they oftentimes will call for the following sugars.

- 100% Maple Syrup
- Raw Agave
- Honey
- Brown Rice Syrup
- Stevia
- Coconut Palm Sugar
- Organic/Vegan Cane Sugar, Brown Sugar and Powdered Sugar

## Flour- (Organic if possible)

- Bob's Red Mill or King Arthur are good brands to purchase and both offer gluten-free options and are non-GMO.
- Unbleached all-purpose flour
- Unbleached white wheat flour
- Wheat flour
- Whole wheat pastry flour
- Garbanzo flour (also known as chickpea flour)
- Coconut flour
- Rice flour
- Sorghum flour
- Tapioca flour- sometimes used for a thickening agent and in gluten-free baking.
- Potato flour- sometimes used for a thickening agent.
- Non-GMO cornstarch

You can blend flours for better nutrition. If a recipe calls for 2 cups of flour for instance, use 1 cup of unbleached all-purpose flour and 1 cup of white wheat flour or whole wheat flour. If you try to use just whole wheat flour you will find your baked goods will come out very dense. Garbanzo flour is interesting to use in baked goods and for making Indian pancakes. Coconut flour, rice flour, sorghum flour, and tapioca flour are used to make a basic gluten free all-purpose flour. There are many chickpea flour cookbooks on the market as well as gluten-free cookbooks, however, many gluten-free baking recipes call for eggs so you will need to replace eggs with one of the alternative egg replacers.

## Other Common Baking Ingredients

Another ingredient you may find a recipe calls for is chocolate chips. Chocolate chips usually have dairy in them. They do make dairy-free vegan chocolate chips and you can find them at some local grocery stores and health food markets. Check the ingredients on the package to be sure they do not contain dairy. Other ingredients, like raisins and cran-raisins, nuts, and seeds are all good in vegan baking. Chatfield's cocoa powder is good and Hershey's cocoa powder is dairy-free.

If a recipe calls for yogurt try So Delicious or Silk non-dairy yogurts. Choose plain and unsweetened yogurt unless a recipe calls for a specific flavor.

Some desserts may call for cream cheese or sour cream. You can find these non-dairy items at your grocery store or check online for recipes using cashews to make your own homemade version of cream cheese and sour cream. They are delicious!

Vinegar may be called for in a baking recipe. You can use organic distilled vinegar or Bragg's Apple Cider vinegar. Making your own "buttermilk" is easy by using any nondairy milk and adding 1 tsp. of lemon juice. For vanilla, be sure to purchase 100% vanilla extract and not imitation. They do make all natural food colorings; however, they are somewhat expensive so I tend not to use them and opt for white or chocolate icings and decorate with fruit toppings, nuts, and seeds. Baking soda and baking powder are necessary ingredients to have on hand for baking; however, be sure your baking powder is *aluminum-free*. Frontier makes organic almond and lemon flavorings sometimes called for in recipes.

Common spices used in baking are ginger, cinnamon, nutmeg, pumpkin, cloves, and allspice.

There are many recipes online, in cookbooks, and on Pinterest that offer really tasty desserts for you to experience. Many stores now carry wholly wholesome pie shells and are available in regular, whole wheat, gluten-free, and spelt and are delicious.

Specialty products such as vegan whipped cream may be found at most health food stores and some local grocery stores. *So Delicious* offers a coconut whip cream made from coconut milk. Soyatoo makes a wonderful whip cream in a can and comes in Soy based and Rice based, both are very good. In earlier chapters, we mentioned silken tofu. Silken tofu works well in pie recipes, puddings, and custards.

The reality with all this information is that you can have desserts and have them taste delicious just by substituting a few ingredients to make far healthier treats for your family. There are no hidden dangers of additives, high fructose corn syrup, and hydrogenated oils that are found on supermarket shelves today that are not only genetically modified but causing ill health and obesity in our children.

Desserts are just that: *desserts* and not meant to be eaten every day. America is obsessed with needing something sweet after every meal. Even though it is healthier to make our own desserts, remember they are still useless calories if consumed on a regular basis. You need to be aware that desserts are meant for celebrating special days, holidays, or events and yes, we all need treats now and then and depriving ourselves from these wonderful tastes can be painful to say the least. Just proceed with caution and consume sweet desserts in moderation. Fresh fruit is our best choice for dessert and most Americans are not eating a single serving of fruit a day. Fresh fruit is a great alternative and by far more beneficial to our bodies!

# Making America Healthy Again!

Lifestyle change is a process that takes most people time to digest and for some, no time at all. Commitment is the first step, then set small goals; this will help you to become more successful in achieving your goals to be healthy. Yes, you will fail now and then and if that happens just pick up where you left off and keep trying. Surround yourself with like-minded people from work or activities you participate in. Having family and friends support your goals for achieving a healthy lifestyle is very important. Begin a yoga class or join a health club. Many states now have meet-up groups where you can engage with like-minded people who are following a vegan plant-based lifestyle offering tips and ideas they use that may help you along your path to better health.

## It's Not a Diet, It's a Lifestyle

The goal here is to have you feeling really good every day! I like this quote by Carl Sandburg: *"It's not that some people have willpower and some don't, it's that some people are ready to change and others are not."*

Remember a plant-based diet, even though called a "diet", is not a diet, it is a *lifestyle change*. It is not meant to be a diet on which you lose weight and then go back to eating all the unhealthy foods you once did. Instead it's a lifestyle change, realizing you are making the right choice to do the right things for your body that will give you optimal nutrition and prevention and keep you on the right path to health and wellness every day. It's not easy at first; it takes determination and a commitment to wanting to be healthy. The best way to start is to begin taking steps to eliminate the foods that are making us sick. You are not going to have to eat less by any means, but just eat right with fresh whole foods instead of "cardboard" processed foods.

We have lived years and years on junk foods and processed foods and over time we have lost touch with what *real* food is and what it can do for our bodies. We have forgotten how good our bodies can actually feel and by that, I mean, we have become so used to not feeling well each morning and throughout our day that it has become the norm in our daily lives.

## Power in Whole Food

There is no diet more powerful than a plant-based diet. There is no diet that will produce results that a plant-based diet can achieve in just a few short weeks or months. Changes begin immediately. No other diet can do this.

It's important to not dwell on the foods you can't eat but embrace the foods that you are so fortunate to be able to consume that are healthy and will nourish your body and mind. Don't let food manufacturers tempt you with foods that will only cause a decline in your health and that of your families. These manufacturers are not concerned with your health and wellness, they are concerned with how much money they can make selling their products to you. It's time we stand up and just say **NO!**

## Taking Control

Our health care cost in America is at an astronomical high and yes, we are all at fault for this. It is time to take responsibility for our eating habits and stop consuming foods that just bring us pleasure without thinking of the consequences of ill health and disease that these foods will bring us down the road. If we continue on the path of eating poorly and not exercising, don't act surprised when illness and disease strikes. It is only a matter of time before it all catches up to us and you fall victim to heart disease, diabetes, or cancer and then expect your doctor to fix it. Yes, we all die, but life can be a blessing and we can enjoy an active life for years if we just make three changes in our life: *eating healthfully, hydrating our bodies, and incorporating moderate exercise.* Strive to make these changes because you love yourself and your body. Don't stay in a negative mode as it will stagnate your life and you will never be able to move forward with health and wellness.

Examine your life today and identify whether your lifestyle is providing optimal health and wellness or sickness and disease and then decide what changes need to take place. If you think about it, a plant-based diet is just common sense. Eating whole foods vs. processed foods and fast foods is not hard to figure out. Food addiction in our nation is at an all-time high. Fast foods (and now super-sizing everything), ice cream, and pastry shops are everywhere and drug stores are needed on every corner to counter the effects these foods create on our health.

Consider this: by the time you pack your family into a car and travel to a restaurant, wait to be seated, wait for a waitress, order your food and drive home again, you can chop a lot of veggies and make a wonderful meal in under 30 minutes and at half the cost. As you begin to eat healthier foods you will be surprised how your taste buds will in fact begin to change and you will actually begin to crave healthier foods rather than unhealthy cravings. Your body begins to eliminate toxins built up in and around your organs and a feeling of wellness begins to take hold. This feeling is so overwhelming that eating clean fresh whole foods will soon be realized as the prescription for which your body was designed.

American appetites are out of control. Fat, sugar, and sodium create enormous pleasure and create a vicious circle from which it is hard to move away from. It is a constant frustration and food addiction that causes more binge eating. When you consume a whole foods plant-based diet you are consuming high fiber foods that curb all of these tendencies. You feel fuller so you are satisfied at each meal which in turns help those who need to lose weight to lose and those who do not need weight loss to easily maintain their weight without any effort.

The sooner you take steps the better. Procrastinating will only delay your efforts in renewed health. Skip all the fad diets and just eat healthfully. You only have one lifetime and one body. Treat your body with love and feed it the nutrients it needs to run optimally as it was designed to do.

## Traditional Medicine & Nutrition

Most of traditional medical industry focuses on treating symptoms and seldom on the cause of disease. We believe that many of today's most devastating diseases are lifestyle-related and may be preventable and often reversible.

Few physicians today receive any significant training in nutrition, natural immune defenses of the body, or how FOOD plays a vital role in our health & wellness. Prevention is one of the KEY factors to *Restoring America's Health* and the foundation of this approach is a healthy nutritional lifestyle.

*Remember Life is short! Enjoy all the things your life has to offer. Be healthy and not sick!*

# Your Health IS Your Wealth!

# Creating Your Own Recipe!

The following recipes are designed to be quick and easy plant-based recipes and allow you to pick and choose vegetables and fruits you and your family most enjoy, as not everyone likes a certain vegetable, spice or herb and some people may be allergic to certain foods. Once you become familiar with plant-based cooking it will be easy for you to recreate your favorite family recipes using plant-based substitutions and experimenting with some of the meat alternatives such as tofu, tempeh, and seitan.

The following dishes are suggested recipes that allow *you* to be the chef! Simply pick and choose your favorite whole grain, vegetables, leafy greens, beans, fruits, nuts, and seeds that you and your family enjoy. These dishes will also work well for divided kitchens where one may be plant-based and others are not. Not everyone in the family is going to want to be plant-based at first. It may take time for others to follow your healthy regime.

*The pictures in this print format book are not in color to save printing and retail cost. For full color pictures, please see our eBook version at a discounted price on Amazon when you purchase the print version.*

- Stir-Fry
- Hummus Wrap
- Burrito
- Pasta Dish
- Salad
- Smoothies
- Pizza
- Veggie Burger
- Soup, Chili or Stew
- Overstuffed Potato, Squash, Tomato, Pepper, Mushroom
- Abundance Bowl-Breakfast, Lunch, or Dinner

# Make a Stir-Fry

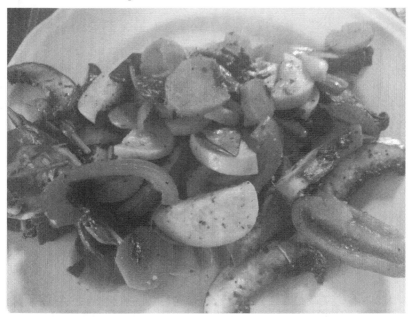

### Preparation
- Equipment needed- Large wok or 12-inch frying pan
- Have all of your vegetable ingredients ready: sliced, diced or shredded. Have all of your liquid ingredients and herbs and spices ready to add to your stir-fry.

### Choose a Protein
Tofu, tempeh, or seitan should be browned first. After browning, set aside. For added flavor you can marinate overnight or an hour or two before you begin your stir-fry. Tofu, tempeh and seitan will pick up the marinated flavors. You can find several different marinades at your local grocery store in your Asian aisle or make your own favorite marinade.

    ☐ **Tofu-** Extra-firm vacuumed sealed. Be sure

to drain twice before slicing or dicing into your stir-fry.

- **Beans** - 1 (15 ounce can) - add beans to your cooked vegetables.
- **Butler Soy Curls**- available online at Butlerfoods.com. Great meat alternative. Soy curls need to be rehydrated in water or marinated before using in recipes.
- **Tempeh**- Tip: Steam your tempeh for 15 minutes. This will release the fermented flavor and make for a nuttier flavor before browning. You can dice, slice, or crumble into your stir-fry.
- **Seitan**- You will find seitan at your health food market or whole foods market. It is located in the cooler section usually next to tofu and comes in a box.

**Choose 3-4 Veggies**
Onions, garlic, and ginger will start your stir-fry with flavor these should be added first before adding your 3-4 vegetables. Be careful that your garlic doesn't burn! Carrots, broccoli, and cauliflower take longer to cook. You can steam them first and then add to your stir-fry last.

- Sweet or green peppers
- Zucchini
- Yellow Squash
- Broccoli
- Cauliflower
- Asparagus
- Brussels Sprouts
- Shredded Cabbage
- Mung Beans- Should be added last as they cook quickly.
- Green Beans
- Snow Peas

- Sugar Snaps
- Shredded Carrots
- Organic Corn
- Carrots
- Onions- red, white, sweet, green
- Garlic
- Fresh Ginger
- Fennel
- Leeks
- Mushrooms- Portobello, white, shiitake, oyster
- Potatoes-sweet, white, red, yellow, purple
- Roma Tomatoes or Sliced Cherry Tomatoes-these types of tomatoes hold up best in a stir-fry and should be added last.

## Choose a Green
You will add your greens as one of your last ingredients as you want them to wilt but not disappear into the dish.
- Bok Choy
- Kale- remove center stem
- Collard- remove center stem
- Spinach
- Swiss Chard- if red remove stem; if white chop and add to stir fry
- Mixed Greens

## Choose a Flavoring
Asian sauces are salty. Avoid adding additional sea salt.
- Soy sauce or Bragg's Liquid Aminos
- Teriyaki Sauce
- Orange Sauce
- Pinch of red pepper flakes
- Pinch of sea salt and black pepper

**Add a Side Dish of Whole Grains**

- Brown Rice- 45-50 minutes. In a hurry? You can use brown rice in a bag. It takes 15-20 minutes to cook.
- Brown Rice Jasmine- 45-50 minutes
- Black Rice- pre-soaked: 20-30 minutes. Dry: 60 minutes
- Wild Rice- 40-45 minutes
- Quinoa- Quick cooking; 20 minutes
- Barley- 45-50 minutes
- Millet- Quick cooking; 20 minutes

Begin by adding a little high-heat oil like *refined* coconut oil (*unrefined* will give your dish a coconut flavor), spectrum canola oil (non-GMO), or grapeseed oil.

For those who are following an oil free diet, just add ¼ cup of water and more as needed. You want to be able to cook your veggies so they are a little crisp on the outside, but not overly cooked and limp. If you're using vegetables that take a longer time to cook such as carrots or potatoes, you can steam them first while preparing your other ingredients for your stir-fry. It is important to have all of your veggies sliced, diced, or shredded before you begin cooking your stir-fry as cooking time goes very quickly. If you have to stop to slice or dice a forgotten vegetable in the middle of cooking others may get overcooked.

**Directions:**
Prepare your whole grains according to package directions. Allow for cooking time so your whole grain is cooked and ready for serving when your stir-fry is complete.

- Steam any vegetables briefly that may take

longer to cook in your stir-fry such as potatoes, broccoli, sliced carrots and cauliflower. Set aside.

- In a wok or 12-inch pan add either ¼ cup of water or 1 T. of oil to your pan. More may be needed as cooking progresses.
- Brown your tofu, soy curls, tempeh, or seitan if using. Set aside after browning.
- Add your garlic, onion, and ginger sauté for approximately 3-5 minutes. Be careful your garlic and ginger do not burn.
- Begin adding your vegetables one at a time and sauté 1-2 minutes, being careful not to overcook them. You want them a little crisp. Add your steamed vegetables into wok.
- Add your beans, tofu, tempeh, or seitan back into stir fry.
- Add your greens and cook just until wilted but not overcooked.
- Add your shredded cabbage at this point if using. If using mung beans, add them last as they cook quickly and always taste better not overcooked but with a little crunch. Add your favorite sauce, remove from heat, and enjoy. Serve alongside your whole grain dish.
- You will find that you can make several different varieties of stir-fry just by changing out the ingredients such as using tofu one day or seitan the next. Just changing your sauce choice will also create a new flavor. There are many great marinades and sauce recipes online.

## Make a Mega Salad

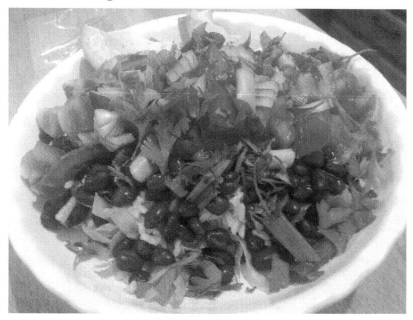

Salads are pretty straightforward. Just add your choice of greens and build from there, being sure to add protein to your salad such as beans, whole grain, nuts, and seeds. Your salad can be greens and veggies or greens and an array of fruit which makes a wonderful breakfast salad.

### Choose Your Greens
- Romaine lettuce
- Mixed Greens- sold in grocery stores in a container
- Arugula
- Spinach
- Kale- remove center stem and tear into pieces. Massage with a little olive oil and sea salt to break down the fibers.
- Sprouts- mung beans, broccoli, radish, sunflower

### Choose a Bean (Protein)

- Chickpeas
- Black Beans
- Kidney Beans
- Pinto Beans
- Red Beans
- White Beans- navy, great northern, cannellini

## Choose a nut or seed
- Walnuts
- Pecans
- Pine Nuts
- Slivered Almonds
- Pistachios
- Pumpkin Seeds
- Sunflower Seeds
- Hemp Seeds
- Sesame Seeds

## Choose several veggies
- Red Onion or Green Onions
- Tomatoes- Cherry or Roma
- Cucumbers
- Cabbage, Red or Green
- Celery
- Corn, fresh or canned (non-GMO organic)
- Carrots, shredded or sliced
- Broccoli
- Cauliflower
- Zucchini
- Yellow Squash
- Yellow, Red, Orange Sweet Peppers
- Jicama root (sweet-tasting like an apple)
- Asparagus

**Choose a Whole Grain - optional as a side dish or mixed in with beans and veggies**

- Brown Rice
- Quinoa
- Buckwheat
- Millet
- Couscous
- Wild Rice
- Wheatberries

**Choose a fruit**

- Pineapple
- Banana
- Apple
- Avocado
- Oranges
- Grapefruit
- Berries- Blueberries, Raspberries, Blackberries
- Grapes- Red or Green

*Add your favorite healthy salad dressing.*
There are several store-bought dressings that are vegan.  Brianna's has several but you need to look for the "V" stamp to see which ones are vegan.  Follow Your Heart makes several vegan creamy salad dressings.  Annie's Organic salad dressings are also a good choice or you can find several vegan salad dressing recipes online. Bragg's makes a wonderful oil-free dressing such as mixed berries and tropical. If making a fruit salad there are many flavors such as strawberry, raspberry, and blueberry.

# Make a Burrito

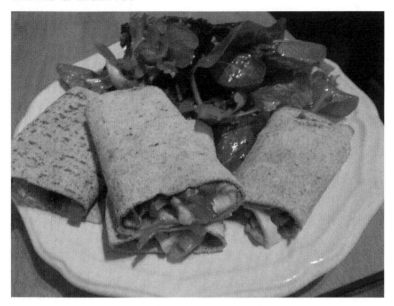

A burrito is a Mexican dish consisting of a tortilla rolled around a filling of beans, whole grains (optional), veggies, tofu or vegan meat alternative such as Gardein chicken strips or Beyond Meat ground crumbles.

**Choose a Healthy Whole Grain Tortilla Wrap** (one without high fructose corn syrup and hydrogenated oils).

**Add a Base Sauce**
- Hummus- Experiment with different flavors!
- Mashed Avocado
- Flavored Mustards
- Vegan Mayonnaise
- Organic Mustard
- Vinaigrette Dressing
- Make an Aioli Sauce- add horseradish and/or garlic to vegan mayo
- Olive Tapenade

- Artichoke pastes
- Hot Sauce

## Choose a whole Grain (precooked)
- Long or short grain brown rice- 45-50 minutes cooking (you can use brown rice in a bag which is now non-GMO and cooks in 15 minutes)
- Jasmine brown rice
- Quinoa- quick cooking
- Millet- quick cooking
- Barley
- Polenta- comes in a roll at your local grocery store look for organic. Simply dice and heat.

## Choose a Protein
- Black bean
- Kidney bean
- Red Bean
- Pinto bean
- White bean
- Garbanzo
- Tofu
- Tempeh
- Seitan
- Soy Curls
- Store bought meat Analogues

## Choose a Green
- Kale
- Spinach
- Mixed Greens
- Romaine Lettuce
- Red Leaf Lettuce
- Butternut Lettuce

## Choose a Veggie- Select 2-3 (dice veggies small)

- Red onion or Green Onion
- Garlic
- Corn, fresh or canned non-GMO organic
- Tomatoes
- Carrots
- Sweet Peppers/green pepper or roasted red peppers
- Jalapeno Peppers
- Broccoli
- Cauliflower
- Zucchini
- Yellow Squash
- Asparagus
- Butternut Squash
- Acorn Squash
- Cucumbers
- Celery
- Edamame (fresh soy beans): these will need to be cooked a little
- Tomatoes- sliced cherry tomatoes
- Artichoke hearts

## Choose a fruit

- Avocado
- Mango

## Add a flavoring

- Lemon Juice
- Lime Juice
- Hot Sauce- Sriracha, Valentina
- Non-Dairy shredded cheese (optional)

## Directions

Add ingredients as follows:

- Tortilla wrap - warmed
- Dressing or sauce
- Greens and veggies and fruit if using such as mangos
- Whole grain- precooked
- Your protein- beans, tofu, soy curls, tempeh, seitan
- To fold the tortilla simply add your ingredients down the center, leaving one end free of filling. Then fold up one end and then fold in both sides and roll.

Note: you can preheat your cooked whole grains, beans, and veggies all together before adding to your tortilla.

# Make a Hummus Wrap

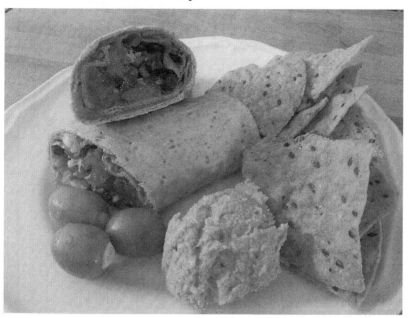

A hummus wrap is similar to a burrito with hummus as a spread with added veggies and meat alternative but can be made using pita bread or bread-free using large lettuce leaves. Pick and choose from the following ingredients.

1. Begin with a tortilla wrap or pita bread or lettuce leaf or green like collard, kale or Swiss chard. (Tip: if using pita bread leave flat like a pizza and fold over instead of filling the inside of pita bread)
2. Spread your favorite blend of hummus on your tortilla, pita bread, or leafy green. (Experiment with different hummus flavors such as artichoke, spinach, roasted red pepper, black bean, edamame, and carrot).
3. Add spinach, shredded romaine lettuce, mixed greens or sprouts.
4. Add sliced tomatoes or cherry tomatoes
5. Shredded carrots
6. Sliced red onion or green onions

7. Add a few sliced black or green olives
8. Add artichoke hearts
9. Add roasted red peppers
10. Add olive tapenade for a Mediterranean wrap
11. Add sweet peppers, broccoli, cauliflower, squash (can be shredded and eaten raw), cucumbers, zucchini, yellow squash, etc.
12. Add your favorite beans
13. Add tofu, tempeh, or seitan- Best to brown a little before adding to your wrap.
14. Add a cooked whole grain- (you can use brown rice in a bag which is now non-GMO and cooks in 15 minutes). quinoa cooks in 20 minutes also.
15. Non-dairy shredded cheese

If using a tortilla, simply fold sides inward and roll up to make a wrap. If using pita bread, lay bread flat and add ingredients and simply fold in half.

Note: You can also change ingredients by adding brown rice or quinoa, beans and sweet peppers. Adding little hot sauce or vinaigrette is also good for flavoring these types of sandwiches.

## Make a Smoothie

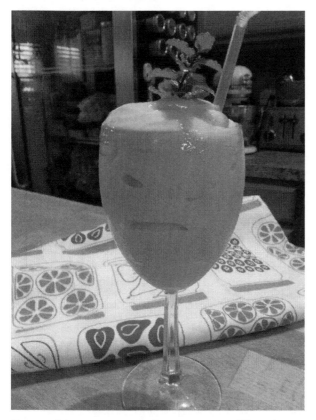

Smoothies are a great way to get fiber into your diet along with vitamins and minerals. You can make smoothie ingredients ahead of time so they are ready to just drop into your blender along with your liquid and have a healthy drink at any time. Making a smoothie only requires combining certain fruits, veggies, and greens that go together well. You can make a fruit smoothie or a vegetable smoothie; however, remember adding greens to either is very important for added health benefits. Here is a list to get you started that you can choose from:

### Fruits, and Berries
- Strawberries
- Blueberries

- Raspberries
- Cranberries
- Cherries
- Grapes
- Kiwi fruit
- Green Apples
- Bananas
- Pineapple
- Mango
- Peaches
- Nectarines
- Pears
- Papaya
- Pomegranate
- Plum

**Melons**
- Cantaloupe
- Honey Dew
- Watermelon

**Citrus**
- Oranges
- Clementines
- Tangelos
- Mandarin
- Lemon
- Lime
- Grapefruit

**Veggies** (making a veggie smoothie)
- Cherry Tomatoes
- Cucumbers
- Celery
- Carrots
- Broccoli

- Summer Squash- Zucchini, yellow squash
- Bell Peppers
- Beets
- Asparagus
- Cherry Tomatoes
- Pumpkin
- Winter Squash

## Greens
- Kale
- Spinach
- Mixed Greens
- Wheat Grass- powder form

## Liquid
- Ice- if fresh fruit and veggies are not already cold or frozen
- Water (filtered is best)
- Coconut Water
- Soy Milk (can be flavored like vanilla)
- Almond Milk (can be flavored like vanilla)
- Rice Milk

## Tea
- White Tea– brew it and cool it. White tea has lower levels of caffeine
- Matcha Tea- Green tea powder
- Hibiscus Tea- high in antioxidant level. It is a caffeine-free herbal tea.

## Other Dry Ingredients
- Oats
- Walnuts
- Chia Seeds
- Flax Seeds
- Hemp Seeds or Powder

- Organic coconut Flakes
- Organic non-dairy protein powder (found online or at health food markets)
- Cocoa powder if you would like a chocolaty drink; just be sure it is dairy-free
- Organic coffee if you would like a coffee flavor
- Powdered Algae- (optional)
  - Spirulina
  - Chlorella
  - Bluegreen Algae

**Sweetness if needed**
- Honey- (some vegans do not consume honey; it is a personal decision)
- Agave
- Medjool Dates
- Maple Syrup
- Stevia

You will find many recipes for smoothies online or on Pinterest. You can use frozen fruit or fresh fruit, citrus, and berries; the choice is yours. Frozen fruit can be expensive but convenient for many. You will find it less expensive to buy fresh fruit and berries and freeze them yourself. Wash your fruit and berries. Chop fruits into chunks and leave berries whole. Place your fruit or berries on a cookie sheet in a single layer, once frozen, place in a plastic freezer bag. This will keep your fruit and berries from sticking together in a clump when frozen.

# Make a Pasta Dish

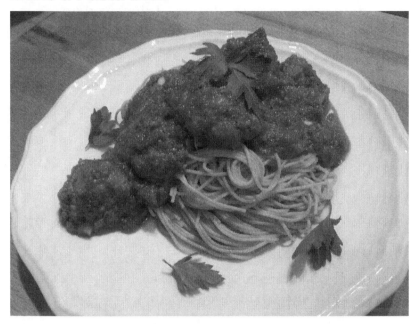

Most of the time we add sauces to our pasta dish; however, there are wonderful recipes that use no sauce and concentrate on adding beans, vegetables, greens, sun-dried tomatoes, olives and touch of extra virgin olive oil for a wonderful pasta meal. If using a sauce, you can also add any of the vegetables and beans mentioned below.

### Choose your 100% Whole Grain Pasta Shape
- Spaghetti
- Linguine
- Penne
- Shells or elbow
- Lasagna
- Orzo
- Rigatoni
- Angle Hair
- Fusilli
- Vegan Ravioli (found at health food markets)

- Asian Noodles- Buckwheat noodles, vermicelli, noodles, Soba noodles, Udon noodles
- Specialty Pasta
  - Gluten Free- Rice, corn, or combination of both
  - Spinach
  - Quinoa
  - Artichoke heart

## Choose your Pasta Sauce
- Marinara
- Mushroom
- Roasted Red Pepper
- Butternut Squash
- Vegan Alfredo- many vegan recipes online using vegan sour cream or cashews for a creamy sauce.
- Canned organic crushed tomatoes to make your own.
- Vegan Pesto made from pine nuts or walnuts
- Asian Noodle Sauces- Soy Sauce, Braggs Liquid Aminos, Teriyaki Sauce, Orange Sauce, Peanut Sauce.

You can use store bought organic sauces but read the ingredient labels to be sure it contains no animal products.

## Choose a Vegetable
- Mushrooms
- Onions
- Garlic
- Sun-dried tomatoes
- Fresh tomatoes
- Sweet peppers
- Olives or olive tapenades
- Artichoke hearts

## Choose a Cheese Alternative if desired

- Daiya, Field Roast, or Follow Your Heart shredded cheese or parmesan cheese
- Tofu Ricotta Cheese-many recipes online.
- Nutritional Yeast (used as a replacement for dairy parmesan cheese)

## Add a Protein

- Meat Free Ground crumbles (Gardein or Beyond Meat) these are gluten-free as well.
- Meat Free Meatballs (Gardein or Beyond Meat) Only Beyond Meat offers gluten-free.
- Vegan Italian sausage is wonderful in Italian dishes; our favorite is Field Roast Brand.
- Add beans to your pasta dishes
- Add crumbled tempeh to your pasta dishes
- Add tofu to your pasta dishes

## Choose a Green to add to your final pasta dish

- Spinach
- Fresh Basil
- Kale
- Swiss Chard
- Arugula

## Choose your Herbs

- Fresh Basil
- Fresh Italian Parsley
- Fresh Cilantro
- Dried herbs: Oregano, Italian seasoning, basil

There are several vegan marinara sauce recipes and tofu ricotta cheese recipes online. Simply Google or search on Pinterest for "Vegan marinara sauces" and "Vegan Ricotta Cheese recipes". There are also nut-based Parmesan cheese recipes to replace dairy Parmesan.

# Make a Pizza

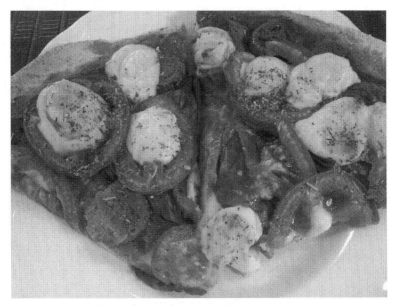

Pizzas are fun to make and delicious. You can make a wonderful pizza without adding all the saturated fat and cholesterol that comes with a pizza you buy at the store or from a pizza shop. We will be using nondairy cheese and replacing meat with any of our meat alternatives such as vegan Italian sausage, vegan ground crumbles, tempeh crumbles, vegan pepperoni or you can substitute with beans and vegetables for a topping. They are easy to make in a jiffy using fresh pizza dough from your super market or you can use whole grain flat bread or pita bread for quick pizzas anytime you want one.

### Choose your whole grain crust
- Store bought fresh pizza dough- preferably whole wheat
- Homemade pizza dough- there are several homemade recipes online and it's so easy to make.
- Whole Grain Flatbread
- Whole Grain Pita Bread

**Choose your Sauce**
- Marinara Sauce
- Pizza Sauce (nondairy)
- Pesto Sauce- Homemade (unless you can find a vegan version at your market without Parmesan cheese in it, but I haven't located one yet).
- Olive tapenades
- If making a Mexican pizza add refried pinto beans as your base in place of marinara or pizza sauce.  Be sure it does not have lard as ingredient.  There are many recipes online for making your own refried beans.

**Choose your Veggie**
- Tomatoes
- Sweet Peppers and Green Peppers
- Mushrooms
- Butternut Squash
- Garlic
- Onions- red, yellow, or green onions
- Zucchini
- Yellow Squash
- Broccoli
- Cauliflower
- Cucumber
- Jalapenos (for Mexican pizza)
- Avocados (for Mexican pizza)
- Corn (for Mexican pizza)
- Artichoke Hearts (Mediterranean pizza)
- Olives (Mediterranean pizza)

**Choose a Green**
- Mixed Greens
- Spinach

- Baby Kale
- Swiss Chard
- Arugula

**Choose a meat substitute (optional)**
- Beans (For a Mexican pizza use Re-fried beans, pinto, or black beans as a base)
- Use white beans for a Mediterranean pizza.
- Tofu
- Tempeh
- Seitan
- Prepackaged alternative meat
  - Ground Crumbles (vegan)
  - Italian Sausage (vegan)
  - Vegan Pepperoni

**Choose a Vegan Cheese (optional)**
- Daiya or Follow Your Heart
- Shredded Mozzarella Cheese- Italian dishes
- Parmesan- Italian dishes
- Cheddar- Mexican Pizza
- Homemade Tofu Feta cheese (recipes online)

Once you have your pizza crust topped with all your ingredients, place in oven at 400-425°F for approximately 15-25 minutes or until cheese topping has melted.

# Make a Veggie Burger

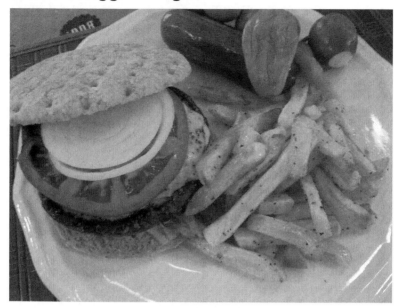

**Choose your Bun.** Be sure to check there is no dairy or egg wash and buy organic if possible.
- Preferably Whole Grain Bun
- Whole Grain Sandwich Thins
- Whole Grain Bagel Thin
- Pita Bread

**Choose your burger.** Check out different brands to find out which one you like the best.
- Gardein Beefless Burger
- Gardein Chipotle Black Bean Burger
- Field Roast Veggie Burgers
- Beyond Meat Beast Burger-Gluten Free
- Amy's Organic Veggie Burger- several varieties that are vegan
- Malibu Garden Burgers
- Sunshine Burgers- Gluten-free- several varieties that are vegan
- Amy's Sonoma Burgers- Gluten-free

- Large Portobello mushrooms are also a replacement for meat burgers and our delicious roasted and topped with all of your favorite fixings.
- Check out recipes online or on Pinterest for homemade burgers made from whole grains and beans. Be sure the recipes are egg-free.

## Choose your Greens
- Spinach
- Mixed Greens
- Baby Kale
- Arugula
- Romaine Lettuce
- Red Leaf Lettuce
- Butter Lettuce
- Only use head lettuce (i.e., iceberg) as a last resort as there is very little nutritional value.

## Choose your veggie
- Onions
- Tomatoes
- Sauerkraut
- Roasted Zucchini and Yellow Squash
- Sautéed Mushrooms
- Cole Slaw (made with vegan mayo) or you can make cole slaw using a vinaigrette dressing.

## Choose your dressing
- Organic Mustard
- Organic Ketchup
- Dairy Free Mayonnaise
- Organic pickle relish
- Pickles

**Choose your Cheese** (optional). Read ingredient labels as some non-dairy cheese may still contain casein, which you want to avoid. Watch for clues such as "lactose-free", which may appear as dairy-free on the package but contains casein, a dairy protein.

- **Daiya** sliced cheese
- **Follow Your Heart** sliced cheese
- **Field Roast** cheese slices

Tip: Veggie burgers, can be baked, grilled, or pan fried on top of the stove.

Looking for the flavor of bacon on your burger? Sauté Portobello mushrooms by marinating your mushrooms in a little liquid smoke, sea salt, and ground black pepper found in most grocery stores. You want them somewhat cooked to release their liquid, but do not burn them. You can also bake them.

## Making a Soup, Chili, or Stew

Soups, chili, and stews are quick and easy and can be made in advance and frozen or have on hand in your refrigerator for those days you may not feel like cooking. It is a great way to finish using vegetables and greens you may have on hand. I like to make a basic vegetable soup that I can add pasta to one day or another day a whole grain like brown rice or quinoa to make it different. Vegan ground crumbles and vegan sausages can be added as well for those who feel the need for a meaty taste and texture in their soups.

**Note:** Omit whole grains such as brown rice or quinoa if making a cream soup.

The following is a checklist you can use to make a delicious soup, stew, or chili. It doesn't matter what you choose as they all go together nicely and you won't be disappointed with the results.

# To Make a Soup

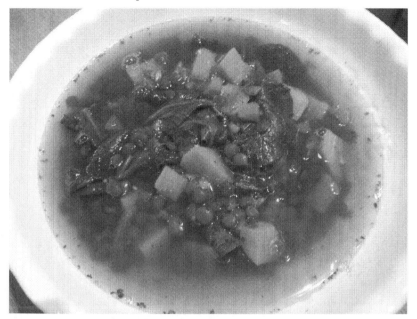

**Choose a Broth** (You will find vegan broths in a cube, paste, or in liquid form or you can make your own homemade vegan broth).

Use 6-8 cups of liquid broth. I have found that 8 cups work better if adding beans or pasta to my soup as they tend to soak up the liquid. Serving size is about 4-6 servings.
- Vegan Vegetable Broth
- Vegan No Chicken Broth- (Imagine is the brand name)
- Vegan No Beef Broth
- Vegan Mushroom Broth

Note: Add 1 T. soy sauce to any broth for more depth of flavor. Some recipes such as curry soups or squash soups may call for canned organic coconut milk.

## Choose a Vegetable
- Zucchini

- Yellow Squash
- Green Beans- fresh or frozen
- Asparagus
- Broccoli
- Cauliflower
- Brussels sprouts
- Sweet peppers
- Green peppers
- Mushrooms
- Onions
- Celery
- Garlic
- Ginger
- Corn
- Edamame- soy beans
- Peas
- Carrots
- Tomatoes- fresh or canned diced tomatoes, or canned fire roasted diced tomatoes
- Cabbage- green or red
- Artichoke Hearts
- Potatoes- All
- Butternut Squash
- Acorn Squash
- Turnips
- Parsnips

## Choose a Green
- Bok Choy- for Asian-type soups
- Swiss Chard
- Collard Greens
- Kale
- Mixed Salad Greens
- Spinach
  Just before your soup is finished, remove from heat, add a handful of chopped greens, and wilt

into your soup being careful not to overcook your greens.

## Choose a Protein
- **Beans-** white beans, black beans, red beds, kidney beans, pinto beans, black eye peas
- **Lentils-** Green lentils will hold up better in soup.
- **Tofu-** You can use either extra firm drained and browned just a little to keep firm and add last to your soup. For Asian soups, you can use silken tofu diced into soups (no draining necessary).
- **Tempeh-** after steaming your tempeh for 15 minutes you can dice or crumble into your soups.
- **Seitan-** If using a vegan sausage or seitan chunks or crumbles I like to brown them just a little before adding to my soups.

## Choose a Whole Grain
- Brown rice- precooked (Quick brown rice you can use brown rice in a bag which is now non-GMO and cooks in 15 minutes)
- Quinoa- precooked
- Buckwheat- precooked
- Wheatberries- precooked
- Barley- precooked
- Millet- precooked
- Asian Noodles- Soba, buckwheat, or udon noodles
- Whole Grain Pasta- you can use any size or shape, even lasagna noodles work well broken into pieces. Note: Many times, I make my soup without a whole grain added right away; that way later you can add a precooked pasta or whole grain to the portion you are just reheating creating a different flavor for mealtime.

## Choose a Spice
Adding spices to your dishes triples the antioxidant

level in all your meals.

- Cumin
- Turmeric
- Paprika
- Cardamom
- Fennel
- Cinnamon
- Allspice
- Cardamom
- Cayenne
- Mint
- Coriander
- Mustard
- Red Pepper Flakes

**Choose a Herb** (dried or fresh)

- Basil
- Rosemary
- Oregano
- Dill
- Cilantro
- Italian Parsley
- Tarragon
- Sage
- Marjoram
- Chives
- Thyme
- Bay Leaf
- Culinary Lavender

# Directions for making soup

- Add a little water (¼ cup) or 1-2 T. of high-heat oil to your pot for sautéing vegetables.
- Add your diced onions and minced garlic
- Add your minced ginger if making an Asian soup
- Add your diced vegetables

- Add your broth- for soup about 6-8 cups.  If adding whole grains, beans or pasta 8 cups of broth is better as they do soak up more liquid.
- Add your protein. Beans, tofu, tempeh, seitan, pasta, or whole grain. If using tofu, tempeh, seitan, or alternative meat product such as Italian sausage or meatballs be sure to brown first and add them back into your soup pot just before serving.
- Add your seasonings – spices and herbs of your choosing.  Italian seasoning is always an easy option- sea salt (not table salt) and black pepper.  Red pepper flakes add a little kick to your soup as well, but do be careful. 1/8- ¼ tsp is plenty.  If you like more heat taste and then adjust the red pepper flakes.
- Bring to a boil and then reduce heat to a low simmer.  Cook until vegetables are tender but not overcooked, if using potatoes or squash be sure to cook until you can pierce a knife through them.  I usually like to add veggies that take longer to cook first such as carrots, potatoes, and squash and then add your other veggies that cook quickly.  If using brown rice, quinoa, or other grain cook separately and then add to your soup pot.

# Making Chili

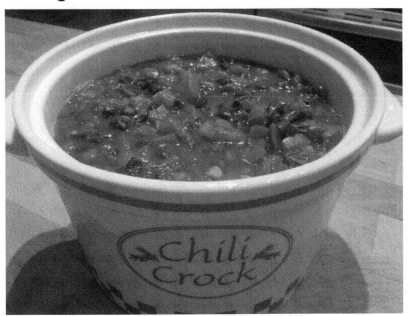

## Broth or Water
- Vegetable Broth
- No-Beef Broth
- No-Chicken Broth
- Mushroom Broth
- ¼-4 cups of Water (optional) add broth or water only if you find it may be too thick and you would like to thin a little.
  *1 T. Soy Sauce or Bragg's Liquid Aminos added to your chili will kick the flavor up a notch!*

## Choose Veggies
- Potato- red, white, sweet-tart
- Onions- red, yellow, green
- Carrots
- Mushrooms (fungi)
- Celery
- Garlic

- Fresh Tomatoes- any
- Canned Crushed Tomatoes
- Canned Diced Tomatoes
- Organic Corn
- Ancho Chilies
- Squash
- Jalapenos
- Canned Green Chilies
- Sweet Red and Yellow Bell Peppers
- Diced Avocado

## Choose a Protein
- Beans- Black bean, red bean, pinto bean, white bean, kidney bean, garbanzo
- Tempeh- crumble after steaming 15 minutes
- Ground Crumbles (Vegan) like Gardein or Beyond Meat
- Lentils

## Choose an Herb
- Thyme
- Oregano
- Cumin
- Chili Powder
- Allspice
- Mexican Chili Powder
- Marjoram
- Fresh Cilantro
- Fresh Italian Parsley
- Mrs. Dash Mixed Seasoning
- 1 ounce of non-dairy unsweetened chocolate
- Sea Salt
- Black Pepper

## Choose from the Following:
- Light Brown Sugar

- Soy Sauce
- Balsamic Vinegar
- Tabasco Sauce
- Adobo Sauce (this is hot, so add a little before adding too much!)

### Choose from these Additional Options
- Lime wedges
- Vegan Sour Cream
- Vegan Shredded Cheese- Daiya or Follow Your Heart Brand

## Three Bean Vegan Chili Recipe

- 1 Tablespoon olive oil
- 1 medium yellow onion, chopped
- 3 garlic cloves, minced
- 28 ounce can of crushed tomatoes (can also use diced)
- 4 ounce can of chopped mild green chilies, drained
- 3 Tablespoons chili powder
- 1 teaspoon cumin
- ½ tsp marjoram
- ½ tsp agave or organic sugar
- 1 can 15.5 ounce black beans drained and rinsed
- 1 can 15.5-ounce great northern or white beans
- 1 can 15.5-ounce dark red kidney beans
- Salt and pepper to taste
- 1 Tablespoon of mixed seasonings (Bragg's)
- Vegan Ground Crumbles (optional)
- Crumbled Tempeh (optional)

Add 1 T. of olive oil (or you can sauté in a little water) to a deep soup pot and sauté onions and garlic, add rest of ingredients, and bring to a boil and simmer on low for 45 minutes. *This is one of my favorite chili recipes; it makes 4-6 servings.*

# Stew

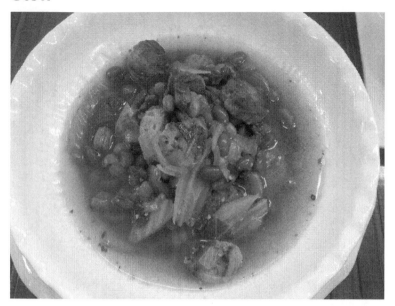

The difference between making a soup or making a stew is how much liquid you are using. A general rule of thumb when making a *soup* is to add 6-8 cups of vegetable broth, whereas in making a *stew* you would use 4 cups of broth. Medium-diced vegetables work best in both stews and soup.

To Make a Stew - *Serving size 4-6*

## Choose your Broth
(4 cups of liquid broth)
- Vegetable Broth
- Mushroom Broth (vegan)
- No Beef Broth
- No Chicken Broth
  Tip: whichever broth you decide to use add 1 Tablespoon of soy sauce to your broth for a savory flavor.

## Choose your Vegetables

- Mushrooms (fungi)- Portobello, shiitake, white button, oyster
- Cauliflower
- Tomatoes- fresh or canned (organic) diced, stewed, fire roasted, crushed
- Broccoli
- Green Beans
- Peas
- Carrots
- Corn
- Fresh Fennel
- Leeks
- Onions
- Artichoke Hearts
- Potatoes
- Squash- butternut, acorn squash (skin removed)
- Eggplant
- Turnips
- Brussels Sprouts
- Cabbage
- Zucchini
- Yellow Squash
- Eggplant
- Garlic
- Fresh Ginger (if Asian stew)

## Choose a Green
- Spinach
- Collard
- Swiss Chard
- Kale

## Choose a Whole Grain
(cook separately and add to pot)
- Brown Rice (Brown rice in a bag which is now non-GMO cooks in 10 minutes)

- Barley
- Quinoa
- Millet
- Buckwheat
- Wheatberries

## Choose a Protein
- Beans- white, red, kidney, pinto, black, black eye peas, garbanzo
- Lentils
- Ground crumbles (vegan) replaces ground round in your recipe
- Tofu
- Tempeh
- Seitan
- Gardein Beefless tips
- Beyond Meat no chicken strips

## Choose a Herb (Fresh or Dried)
- Rosemary
- Thyme
- Oregano
- Parsley
- Basil
- Sage
- Italian Seasoning

## Directions:
1- Add a ½ cup of water to your soup pot or 1-2 T. of high-heat oil.
2- Add your chopped onion. Cook until translucent.
3- Add your minced garlic. 1-3 Tsp.
4- Add your desired diced Vegetables. Cook another 5 Minutes adding a little more water so as not to burn if needed.
5- Add your vegetable broth and 1 T. soy sauce for a rich flavor.

6- Add your seasonings
7- Bring to a boil and then simmer until vegetables are tender but not overcooked.
8- Add in your protein such as beans or browned tofu, tempeh, seitan, or other alternative meat product.
9- Add in your cooked grain
10- Add your choice of greens and cook just until wilted.

# Overstuffed Potato, Squash, Tomato, Pepper or Mushroom

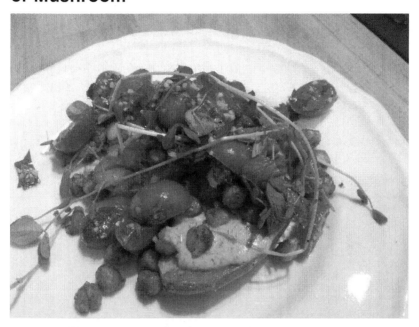

A general rule of thumb when stuffing a potato is to use vegetables, greens, and beans. When stuffing a vegetable like sweet peppers or squash, use a precooked whole grain, such as brown rice, quinoa, or barley mixed with other small diced veggies from the list below. Adding an alternative meat such as vegan Italian sausage, ground crumbles, or your favorite bean will add more flavor and texture to your recipe.

**Choose Your Base for Stuffing**
- Potato- sweet potato or russet potato
- Squash- large zucchini, large yellow squash, acorn Squash, pumpkin, butternut squash, spaghetti squash
- Tomato, large
- Avocado, large
- Green Pepper
- Red Pepper

- Yellow Pepper
- Orange Pepper
- Mild Poblano Pepper- (Mexican flair)
- Portobello Mushrooms- Look for large size

*This list gives you 10 different meals for your family to enjoy just by changing your base vegetable to stuff!*

## Choose a Whole Grain
- Brown rice- long grain or short grain- (Brown rice in a bag which is now non-GMO and cooks in 10 minutes)
- Jasmine brown rice
- Quinoa
- Buckwheat
- Barley
- Millet
- Wheatberries

## Choose a Vegetable
- Broccoli
- Cauliflower
- Artichoke hearts
- Tomatoes
- Shredded carrots
- Onions- Red, White, Sweet, Green

## Choose a Protein
- Beans- dried or canned
- Tofu- use extra-firm vacuumed sealed and drain twice before browning
- Butler Soy Crumbles (available online at Butlerfoods.com)
- Tempeh- Steam 15 minutes before marinating and browning
- Seitan Vegan Crumbled Grounds- brown before

adding to your filling
- Seitan Vegan Sausages- brown before adding to your filling

*If using a meat alternative, I always like to dice and brown them first before adding to the filling you are using.*

## Choose a fresh or dried herb
- Rosemary
- Thyme
- Oregano
- Parsley
- Basil
- Sage
- Italian dried Seasoning

## Choose a Non-Dairy Cheese (optional)
- Shredded Mozzarella
- Shredded Cheddar
- Vegan Sour Cream
  *Daiya or Follow your Heart Brand suggested.*

## Directions:
Begin by choosing which vegetable you will be stuffing. If you are using a white baked potato I find adding steamed vegetables like carrots, broccoli, and cauliflower, greens, and beans are a great topping. You can also add a dab of vegan sour cream on top.

Sweet potatoes go well with chickpeas, greens, and veggies with hummus dressing. Roasted vegetables and chickpeas seasoned with cumin, paprika, and cinnamon are wonderful.

## Hummus Dressing Recipe
- ¼ cup of your favorite hummus

- 2-3 T. lemon juice
- A little water and thin to a dressing consistency

If you are stuffing a zucchini, pepper, squash, tomato, etc. I like to use a whole grain topping mixed with chopped onions, garlic, vegan Italian sausage, beans, and spices or herbs. You want to flavor your whole grain and then stuff your vegetable and top with a vegan shredded cheese if you desire. If you're making a Mexican topping, hot sauce is always a nice addition. If you're making a Mediterranean stuffing, you can use a vinaigrette dressing.

# Make an Abundance Bowl

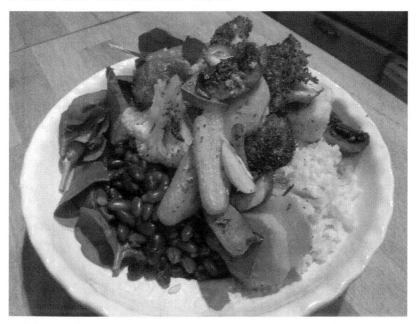

When I discovered how to make abundance bowls (also known as Buddha bowls and nourishment bowls), I fell in love with the idea and how easy they were to make, but most importantly how nutritious they were! Abundance bowls create a power plate that uses our four food groups such as protein, vegetables, whole grains, and fruit all in one dish. They are good any time of the day as you can make it a fruit abundance bowl for breakfast or vegetable abundance bowl for lunch or dinner. They also make a convenient meal to take to work. Abundance bowls can be made Mediterranean, Asian, Italian, Indian, and Mexican.

It offers the best in plant-based cuisine. When adding vegetables for this type of bowl it is best to steam or roast. Beans such as chickpeas are great roasted or sautéed with a little cumin, paprika, cinnamon, sea salt, and black pepper. Greens such as Swiss chard, kale or collard are best steamed or sautéed in a little water with garlic, sea salt, and black pepper.  Steamed baby bok choy versus larger leaves are best for abundance bowls.  Choose a good-sized bowl for each person.  Many Asian markets sell beautiful bowls that work perfectly for abundance bowls.

## Choose Your Green
- Fresh Greens
  - Shredded Romaine Lettuce
  - Mixed Greens
  - Broccoli Rabe
  - Spinach- You can either wilt or keep as is and add to bottom of bowl.
- Wilted Greens
  - Kale- Wilt until tender
  - Swiss Chard- Wilt until tender
  - Collard Greens- Wilt until tender
  - Bok choy- Wilt until tender

Wilted Greens will always be added to the top or side of each bowl.

## Choose your Vegetables
- Broccoli
- Cauliflower
- Green Beans
- Carrots
- Asparagus
- Tomatoes- Fresh, canned diced, fire roasted
- Cucumbers
- Eggplant
- Sweet Peppers
- Green Peppers
- Cucumbers
- Fennel
- Onions
- Leeks
- Olives

- Daikon Radish
- Burdock Root
- Mushrooms (fungi)
- Beets
- Zucchini
- Yellow Squash
- Acorn Squash
- Butternut Squash
- Corn
- Peas
- Snow Peas
- Sugar Snap Peas
- Garlic
- Ginger

## Choose your Whole Grain
- Brown Rice- Long or Short grain- (Quick brown rice you can use brown rice in a bag which is now non-GMO and cooks in 15 minutes)
- Quinoa
- Buckwheat
- Millet
- Wheatberries
- Polenta
- Barley

## Choose a Pasta - *Optional*
- 100% Whole wheat pasta- any size or shape
- Artichoke flour Pasta
- Quinoa Pasta- Gluten Free
- Rice Pasta- Gluten Free
- Buckwheat pasta- Good in Asian Dishes
- Soba Noodles – Good in Asian Dishes
- Udon Noodles- Good in Asian Dishes
- Vermicelli Noodles- Good in Asian Dishes

**Choose your Protein**

- Beans- Chickpeas, Black Beans, Kidney Beans, Red Beans, Mung Beans, Pinto Beans
- Tofu- extra-firm drained twice and browned until golden on the outside.
- Seitan- I like to brown a little. You can add your favorite sauce such as teriyaki or orange sauce for additional flavor to seitan.
- Tempeh- Steam 15 minutes before marinating with your favorite sauce and browning.
- Gardein product vegan chicken strips- You will want to brown or bake these first.
- Gardein product beefless tips- You will want to heat through on top of stove or oven.
- Vegan Italian Sausage- You will want to brown first.
- Vegan Meatballs- You will want to brown first.
- Non-Dairy Greek yogurt (breakfast bowls)

**For a Breakfast Bowl - Choose a Fruit, Citrus or Berry**

- Mango
- Kiwifruit
- Oranges
- Grapefruit
- Strawberries
- Raspberries
- Blueberries
- Blackberries
- Apple
- Peaches
- Nectarines
- Pears
- Banana
- Pineapple

Tip: Ingredients that go well in a breakfast abundance bowl are brown rice or quinoa, non-dairy yogurt (plain or flavored), nuts and seeds, and chopped spinach with a drizzle of honey or agave syrup. Try a berry and banana combination or citrus and banana combination.

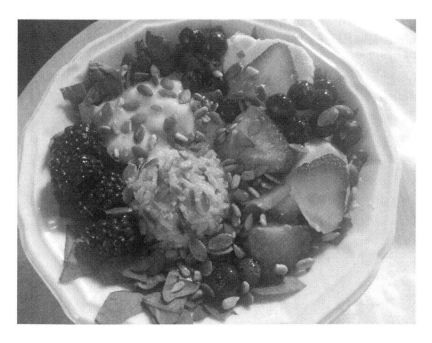

## Choose a Nut and Seed
- Pine Nuts
- Slivered Almonds
- Pecans
- Walnuts
- Cashews
- Peanuts
- Sunflower seeds
- Pumpkin Seeds
- Chia Seeds
- Hemp Seeds

## Choose Your Seasonings

*You can use dried or fresh herbs and spices*
- Rosemary
- Thyme
- Oregano
- Parsley
- Basil
- Cilantro
- Sage
- Fresh Italian Parsley
- Fresh Basil
- Fresh Cilantro
- Turmeric
- Paprika
- Cinnamon
- Cardamom
- Fennel Seeds
- Cumin
- Garlic
- Ginger

## Choose your Dressing
- Vegan Sour Cream and hot sauces- Mexican bowls
- Hummus dressing
- Avocado dressing
- Asian Sauces- Teriyaki sauce or Peanut sauce
- Balsamic Vinegar for Italian bowls

## Dressings, Sauces & Condiments

You can use any of your favorite vegan dressings; however, making your own is easy to do especially in a pinch. One of our favorites is made using hummus. Hummus comes in many flavors now: garlic, roasted red pepper, black bean, artichoke, and even carrot. Here is an easy recipe for a salad dressing that pairs well with abundance bowls.

### *Hummus Salad Dressing*
¼ cup of your favorite hummus
2-3 Tablespoons of fresh lemon juice
add a little water to mix to dressing consistency

If you are making a **Mexican** abundance bowl add a hot sauce for your dressing. A favorite of ours is *Valentina Hot Sauce.*

If you are making a **Mediterranean** abundance bowl, try *Brianna's French Vinaigrette* or use Herb de Provence salad dressing. Be sure to read ingredients to ensure that they are vegan.

Hummus or avocado dressings pair well with **Asian** abundance bowls. You can find many homemade vegan salad dressing recipes online with Google search.

If you are making a **fruit** abundance bowl I like to use either Bragg's tropical or mixed berry no-oil dressings or Brianna's vegan strawberry salad dressings. You can also use your favorite honey drizzled onto your fruit, whole grain, and non-dairy yogurt. If you are a vegan who does not consume honey they do make a vegan version of honey made from apples or you can substitute maple syrup, agave syrup, or flavored brown rice syrup which comes in strawberry or blueberry flavors. Vegan Honey- is by Bee Free Honey and Flavored Brown Rice Syrup- Suzanne Specialties.

# What to Eat for Breakfast?

We have covered several ideas for lunch and dinners that are quick and easy to make and will get you started easily on a plant-based diet. I am sure you're wondering what you can eat for breakfast. You are never without a healthy option for breakfast. You can make it as simple as you want or more savory, in less than 30 minutes. There are recipes galore online and on Pinterest to help get you started just by entering vegan breakfast ideas.

I hope to get you started with a few ideas:

## Quick and Easy Breakfast

When time is short and you're in a hurry

- **Fruit or Green Smoothie**
- **Organic Old Fashion Oats**- Hot or Cold (make your own ready to go granola). Add a tablespoon of peanut butter or flavor your cooked oats with organic pumpkin puree.
- **Whole Grain Waffles**- Top with a fresh berry compote or organic maple syrup, brown rice syrup, or agave syrup.
- **Whole Grain Pancakes**- Make ahead of time and freeze so they are ready to reheat. Add your favorite berries, and if you desire a sweetener add a little organic maple syrup, brown rice syrup, or agave syrup.
- **Parfait with Non-dairy Yogurt**- Layer your parfait by adding organic oats, nuts, seeds, berries, and your favorite non-dairy yogurt.

Remember you can also make a non-dairy yogurt parfait or raw oat cereal and place in a mason jar to take with you to work if time is of the essence in the morning. Bring your smoothie in an insulated mug.

## Savory Breakfast

When you have a little more time in the morning.

## Tofu Scramble

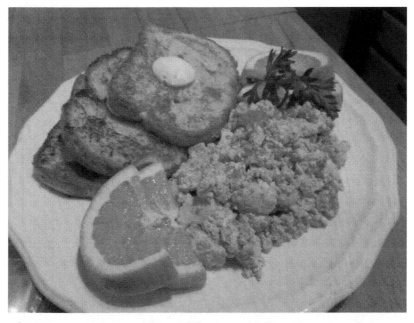

These are easy to make. I like to use firm or extra-firm vacuumed-sealed tofu for my scramble. Remember you will need to empty the liquid from the box and press the tofu a second time to release the added water in the tofu itself. I would recommend doing the second press the night before and place in the refrigerator. Your tofu will be perfect and ready to go in the morning.

Once your tofu is pressed you can either dice it or crumble it. If crumbling be sure to not crumble too small; leave it in what I call "egg-sized" scramble pieces. Place your tofu in a dish and add ¼ tsp. Of turmeric and 1/2 tsp. Of Kala Namak black salt (This salt is actually pink in color but not to be confused with Himalayan pink salt which is also pink. Kala Namak black salt consists mostly of sodium chloride which gives it a sulfuric egg smell and taste when using tofu as your egg replacer in dishes like tofu scramble or omelets). Set bowl aside while you prepare any vegetables you would like to add to your tofu scramble.

## Choose your Veggies
- Mushrooms
- Red, white, or green onions
- Cherry tomatoes
- Sweet Peppers
- Green Peppers
- Jalapenos for Mexican fair
- Asparagus
- Broccoli
- Garlic

Add 1 T. of oil to your sauté pan (or if oil-free add ¼ cup of vegetable broth or water to your pan). Sauté your choice of vegetables until just tender. Set aside. Add your tofu scramble into sauté pan and, using a spatula, carefully mix the tofu until heated through and the turmeric is mixed into the tofu and turns the color to an even yellow. Add your diced cooked veggies and handful of greens back into pan. Heat through and serve. Turn onto a plate and serve alongside any alternative breakfast sausage or try hash browns or sliced potatoes as a side dish.

## Choose a Green
- Spinach
- Kale
- Italian Parsley
- Cilantro

Don't forget to add spices and fresh herbs of your choice. Adding salsa or hot sauce is another idea for a Mexican Scramble.

# Potato Hash

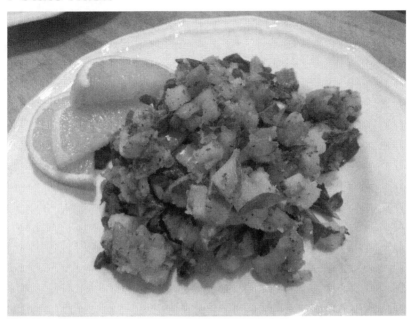

This happens to be another great savory dish you can enjoy for breakfast. You can use either hash browns or diced potatoes (white or sweet potatoes); they both work well. It is best to steam or roast your diced potatoes before adding to your sauté pan. Sauté any vegetables you like such as zucchini, yellow squash, sweet peppers, onions, and garlic or other diced vegetables of your choosing and sauté until tender. Add your steamed potatoes to the veggies. Add seasonings of your choice along with a handful of your favorite greens and heat another 2-3 minutes until your greens have slightly wilted and serve. If using shredded potatoes, I like to brown them a little first and then add in my veggies. If adding your favorite meat alternative such as Italian, apple or sage vegan sausage, or vegan ground crumbles, I like to brown these first as well then add in my vegetables and potatoes. This is a hearty breakfast that won't disappoint family members!

# Breakfast Burrito or Tortilla Wrap

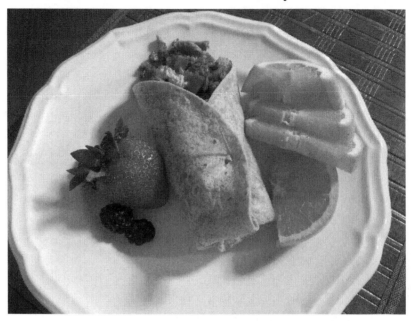

These are delicious and kids will love them! You can begin with your favorite brand of tortilla or you can use whole grain pita bread (be sure they are the larger size for this). Next add your favorite hummus or mash an avocado with a little lemon juice for your foundation. Add your greens; spinach or prepackaged mixed greens are best. Next cook your diced onions and sweet red, yellow, orange, or green peppers and set aside. Next brown any meat alternative you would like to use such as Italian sausage or ground crumbles and set aside (you can also use beans in place of meat alternative). Next make a tofu scramble. Mix your cooked veggies in with your tofu scramble. Lastly add your cooked meat alternative or beans on top of your greens. Add your tofu scramble next and fold your tortilla or pita bread and enjoy. Hot sauce is very good as a final topping!

# Healthy Snack Ideas

Snacking is a way of life, let's face it! Unhealthy processed foods in the supermarket have taken over our lives and now it is time to replace unhealthy snacks with healthier options. Here are a few suggestions that are healthy and will satisfy any cravings for an in-between meal snack attack!

1. Fresh fruit is always available and easy to transport.
2. Handful of nuts or seasoned roasted nuts are delicious!
3. Vegetables and Hummus Dip (celery, carrots, zucchini, yellow squash, radishes, broccoli, cauliflower, raw asparagus, cucumbers). Hummus dip and avocado dips are now available in small packets to easily carry with you to work.
4. Apple slices spread with nut butters and topped with chopped nuts or seeds
5. Air-popped popcorn with cheesy nutritional yeast
6. Seasoned roasted chickpeas
7. No bake energy bars or cookies- Many recipes online or on Pinterest
8. Yonanas ice cream machine- makes delicious ice cream using just fresh fruit, no sugar.
9. Make non-dairy yogurt and fruit popsicles
10. Frozen bananas dipped in dark chocolate and crushed nuts and seeds
11. Tofu-banana vegan chocolate pudding:

- 2 boxes of "silken" firm or extra firm tofu
- 3 ripe bananas
- 1 cup vegan chocolate chips, melted
- 1 tsp. of pure vanilla extract

Blend all ingredients and pour into individual cups and place in refrigerator until firm. You can top your pudding with So Delicious Coconut whipped non-dairy topping and diced strawberries.

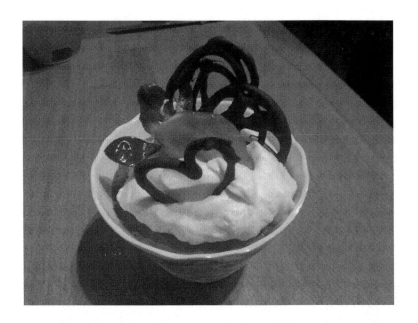

12. Nut Butter and Jam Banana wraps- Spread your favorite peanut butter or nut butter on your whole grain tortilla, add your favorite jam, and one whole banana and roll up the tortilla.

13. Mix diced apples and red grapes with peanut butter, add a drizzle of honey, and add to butter lettuce leaves and roll up.

14. Freeze your favorite non-dairy yogurt. Make a slice in the top of the container and place a popsicle stick in the center before freezing.

15. Make a smoothie

All of these snack ideas will keep you on a path to good nutrition. It will become easier to avoid all the temptations at the store once you begin to feel the effects of clean eating. It is the food choices you make today that will determine your health tomorrow.

# Smart Phone Apps

Smart phone apps help us to find restaurants that are vegan, vegan-friendly or even grocery stores that offer us vegan options if traveling out of town.

A good app for your Smart Phone is called *"Happy Cow"* which is a free download and will show vegan and vegan-friendly restaurants in whatever location you may be, as well as health markets and stores that carry vegan products. It's especially handy if you're traveling out of your state. If you don't have a smart phone you can still check for vegan restaurants and stores on their website at HappyCow.net

If you're traveling by car and have neither a smart phone or computer handy, these restaurants serve vegan options: Chipotle, which offers a vegan tofu sofritos rice bowl that is delicious; Subway and Panera Bread offer a vegetable sub or sandwich. Need a breakfast? Ask for a potato veggie scramble in place of eggs and be sure they don't use butter or cheese on it. It may seem difficult at first, but as you get used to eating healthfully, eating out and recognizing dishes that are meat-, fish-, dairy- and egg-free becomes easier and you will soon find yourself able to adjust a restaurant meal by omitting the animal protein and still have it taste wonderful.

Restaurants are getting better and usually will have one entree or two that you can choose or adjust by leaving out certain ingredients like cheese or meat. Italian restaurants offer spaghetti with marinara sauce and sometimes they have a vegan mushroom ravioli with marinara sauce. Thai restaurants and Asian restaurants have vegetable dishes free of animal products and are delicious. Some Mexican restaurants can accommodate vegans; you can always call ahead of time to be sure or remember: many of their menus are online now.

Not all restaurants have veggie burgers on their menu, but if you ask they oftentimes have them. If you're traveling on the road, it's always a good idea to bring your lunch with you just in case you can't find a healthy restaurant. Some roadside gasoline stops are now offering fresh fruit and of course you can always find a healthy bag of nuts and seeds to go with your fruit.

Another good app for your smart phone is called *"Fooducate"*. This app is used in your grocery store allowing you to scan a product for its health benefit before you buy the product. It will grade the product from A to F and will tell you if there are hidden ingredients that may not be vegan in the product that you may have missed and whether the product contains genetically modified ingredients. It is a great app!

# What Is YOUR Lifestyle?

Lifestyle change is completely up to you. It can't be decided for you by someone else. It is a choice of whether you want to live a healthy life into your golden years or you settle for sickness and feeling miserable day in and day out stemming from bad food choices and lack of exercise. Ask yourself if being a couch potato is worth the health consequences of disease and illness? Walking just 30 minutes each day will make such a difference in your health. A simple walk can lower your blood pressure, regulate your blood sugar, and get your heart pumping.

It seems becoming healthy is something we set aside in life until the inevitable happens like illness. We have become so indoctrinated by TV ads that a pill will make us better in no time and a Big Mac is healthier than fresh vegetables and fruit. We are persuaded by manufacturers that processed foods are healthy foods and eating steak, chicken, and pork is good for us, while research has confirmed meat has no nutritional value, lacking in any fiber, and injuring our bodies with unnecessary saturated fat and cholesterol. It should seem very clear to us that a whole foods diet would be far better and more nutritional for our health in the long run.

Attitudes play a big role in healthy eating. If you truly believe you can't live without certain unhealthy foods, then by all means, continue with the Standard American Diet, but if you want and have a real desire to live and thrive I encourage each and every one of you to take a thirty-day challenge eating a 100% whole foods plant-based diet and compare the two.

Eating a whole foods plant-based diet does take commitment and as stated earlier it doesn't have to be accomplished overnight. Eliminating unhealthy foods by taking small steps over time will make you more successful in achieving a healthy goal. Don't be discouraged if you fail; just start again.

As with any new challenge, it takes practice and time. There is no downside to a plant-based diet. You will only find renewed health and wellness. Living life healthy, not sick, and enjoying all the beauty we are blessed with in nature to experience daily should be our goal and priority in life.

Now is the time to tear up your bucket list because now you will have all the time in world to be healthy and alive and time to experience all that life has to offer! A healthy lifestyle is yours for the taking if you simply watch what you're putting on your plate.

# *It's That Simple!*

# About the Author

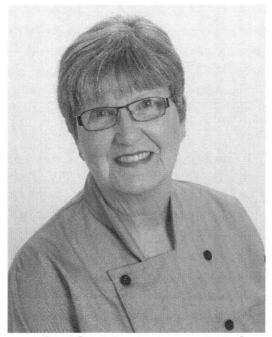

## Chef Nancy A. Stein
**Owner of Whole Foods 4 Healthy Living**
**Orlando, Florida USA**
http://www.wholefoods4healthyliving.com/

Chef Nancy Stein is a plant-based chef based in Orlando, Florida. She creates and offers new and delicious plant-based cuisine and recipes that are both healthful and delicious. With a focus on health & wellness, Nancy has been serving the central Florida area through her company Whole Foods 4 Healthy Living for over seven years.

Nancy received her Certificate in Plant Based Nutrition from eCornell University under a program developed by Dr. T. Colin Campbell. Prior to her work in the field of nutrition and health, Nancy served with Delta Airlines in many capacities for over a period of 25 years. Her experiences included working as a flight attendant, reservations, ticketing, baggage service and hostess in the premier Delta Crown Rooms in Detroit and Orlando. She understands the stresses and challenges found in all workplaces and how it can impact diet and lifestyle choices.

Working closely with her husband, Skip Stein, a Nutritional Holistic Prostate Cancer Survivor, she has worked diligently to promote a Plant-Based Lifestyle approach to support disease reversal and prevention.

Through her classes on Plant-Based Cuisine, Chef Nancy has trained many people how to adopt healthier lifestyle choices. The Corporate Wellness Program is focused on business communities and offers programs to promote both health, wellness, and productivity.

■■■■■■■■■■■■■■■■■■■■■■■■■■■■■■■■■■■■■■■■■■■■■■■■

Made in the USA
San Bernardino, CA
29 December 2017